Pediatric Emergency Ultrasound

Pediatric Emergency Ultrasound
A Concise Guide

Lead Editors
Marsha A. Elkhunovich, MD
Tarina L. Kang, MD

Associate Editors
Courtney Brennan, MD
Kathryn Pade, MD

Contributing Authors
Rashida Campwala, MD
Jessica Rankin, MD
Kristin Berona, MD

Illustrations by
Courtney Brennan, MD

Children's Hospital Los Angeles
Division of Emergency and Transport Medicine
Keck Hospital and Keck School of Medicine
University of Southern California
and
Los Angeles County + University of Southern California
Medical Center
Department of Emergency Medicine
Los Angeles, California

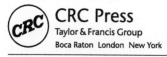

CRC Press
Taylor & Francis Group
Boca Raton London New York

CRC Press is an imprint of the
Taylor & Francis Group, an **informa** business

First edition published 2020
by CRC Press
6000 Broken Sound Parkway NW, Suite 300, Boca Raton, FL 33487-2742

and by CRC Press
2 Park Square, Milton Park, Abingdon, Oxon, OX14 4RN

© 2020 by Taylor & Francis Group, LLC

CRC Press is an imprint of Taylor & Francis Group, an Informa business

This book contains information obtained from authentic and highly regarded sources. While all reasonable efforts have been made to publish reliable data and information, neither the author[s] nor the publisher can accept any legal responsibility or liability for any errors or omissions that may be made. The publishers wish to make clear that any views or opinions expressed in this book by individual editors, authors or contributors are personal to them and do not necessarily reflect the views/opinions of the publishers. The information or guidance contained in this book is intended for use by medical, scientific or health-care professionals and is provided strictly as a supplement to the medical or other professional's own judgement, their knowledge of the patient's medical history, relevant manufacturer's instructions and the appropriate best practice guidelines. Because of the rapid advances in medical science, any information or advice on dosages, procedures or diagnoses should be independently verified. The reader is strongly urged to consult the relevant national drug formulary and the drug companies' and device or material manufacturers' printed instructions, and their websites, before administering or utilizing any of the drugs, devices or materials mentioned in this book. This book does not indicate whether a particular treatment is appropriate or suitable for a particular individual. Ultimately it is the sole responsibility of the medical professional to make his or her own professional judgements, so as to advise and treat patients appropriately. The authors and publishers have also attempted to trace the copyright holders of all material reproduced in this publication and apologize to copyright holders if permission to publish in this form has not been obtained. If any copyright material has not been acknowledged please write and let us know so we may rectify in any future reprint.

Except as permitted under U.S. Copyright Law, no part of this book may be reprinted, reproduced, transmitted, or utilized in any form by any electronic, mechanical, or other means, now known or hereafter invented, including photocopying, microfilming, and recording, or in any information storage or retrieval system, without written permission from the publishers.

For permission to photocopy or use material electronically from this work, access www.copyright.com or contact the Copyright Clearance Center, Inc. (CCC), 222 Rosewood Drive, Danvers, MA 01923, 978-750-8400. For works that are not available on CCC please contact mpkbookspermissions@tandf.co.uk

Trademark notice: Product or corporate names may be trademarks or registered trademarks, and are used only for identification and explanation without intent to infringe.

ISBN: 978-1-138-33239-3 (hbk)
ISBN: 978-1-138-33228-7 (pbk)
ISBN: 978-0-429-44665-8 (ebk)

Typeset in Minion Pro
by Nova Techset Private Limited, Bengaluru & Chennai, India

Contents

Introduction	vii
Ultrasound probes	ix

PART I　CIRCULATORY SYSTEM　　1

1　Cardiac	3
2　Inferior vena cava	13

PART II　RESPIRATORY SYSTEM　　19

3　Pulmonary	21

PART III　MUSCULOSKELETAL SYSTEM　　33

4　Long bone	35
5　Clavicle	43
6　Shoulder	49
7　Elbow	53
8　Hip	61
9　Knee	67
10　Ankle	75

PART IV　INTEGUMENTARY SYSTEM　　81

11　Soft-tissue	83
12　Neck	93

PART V　DIGESTIVE SYSTEM　　103

13　Appendix	105
14　Intussusception	111
15　Pylorus	117
16　Biliary	121

PART VI TRAUMA — 131

17 Focused assessment sonography in trauma (FAST) — 133

PART VII RENAL, URINARY, AND REPRODUCTIVE SYSTEMS — 145

18 Renal — 147
19 First trimester pregnancy — 157
20 Testicular — 165

PART VIII PROCEDURAL — 171

21 Femoral nerve block — 173
22 Intraosseous placement — 179
23 Lumbar puncture — 183
24 Endotracheal tube confirmation — 189
25 Peripheral intravenous placement — 193
26 Upper extremity nerve blocks — 199
27 Central line placement — 207

PART IX NERVOUS SYSTEM — 213

28 Ocular — 215

Bibliography — 223
Index — 231

Introduction

Point-of-care ultrasound (POCUS) has been used to improve patient care for over 35 years. POCUS had its beginnings in the 1980s, when it was used as a bedside modality to determine the presence of hemo-peritoneum in trauma patients. Since then, the extent to which POCUS has influenced the way clinicians evaluate patients has been profound, so much so that by 1990, the American College of Emergency Physicians (ACEP) introduced the first POCUS practice statement. In 2001, the Accreditation Council for Graduate Medical Education (ACGME) mandated ultrasound training for Emergency Medicine residents who practice in the United States. Given its success as a reliable and safe bedside modality, the use of POCUS in a variety of emergency clinical presentations is considered standard-of-care.

It is no wonder that the use of POCUS quickly took root in pediatric emergency medicine, given the safety of ultrasound technology, the desire to decrease radiation exposure in children, and the inherent difficulty of assessment of pediatric patients. A survey done in 2011 demonstrated that 95% of Pediatric Emergency Medicine fellowship programs in the United States utilize point-of-care ultrasound, and 88% provide some degree of training for their fellows (Marin JR, et al. *J Ultrasound Med.* 2012; 31:1357–1363.). In 2015, the American Academy of Pediatrics (AAP) issued the first pediatric-specific ultrasound guidelines and ultrasound training has now been incorporated into several pediatric specialty-training programs.

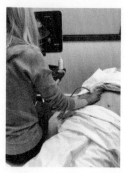

This book was developed as a learning tool and a quick reference for practitioners who take care of children in both emergent and non-emergent settings. We hope this handbook will help pediatric providers enhance the assessment of their patients, allow more efficient diagnosis and treatment, and improve procedural safety and comfort.

Happy scanning

Marsha A. Elkhunovich, MD
Tarina L. Kang, MD

Ultrasound probes

5-1 MHz low-frequency phased array transducer

Uses:

- Renal US
- FAST
- Focused echocardiogram
- Focused biliary

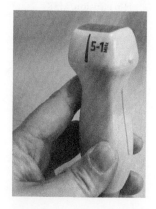

15-6 MHz High-frequency linear transducer

Uses:

- US-guided lumbar puncture
- US-guided peripheral vascular access
- Intraosseous line confirmation
- Hip effusion/MSK
- Soft-tissue infection
- Appendicitis US
- Intussusception US
- Pylorus US
- Ocular
- Lung pleura

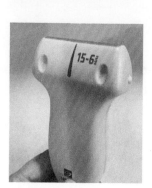

5-2 MHz curvilinear transducer

Uses:

- Appendicitis US (larger BMI)
- Lung US (older children)
- Renal
- FAST
- Biliary
- Hip effusion/MSK
- Gyn/Pregnancy

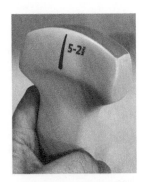

P10X 4-8 MHz transducer

Uses:

- Neonatal head
- Abdominal
- Focused echocardiogram

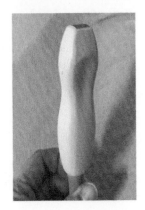

CX11 8-5 MHz transducer

Uses:

- Abdomen
- Nerve and musculoskeletal
- Vascular access
- Focused echocardiogram

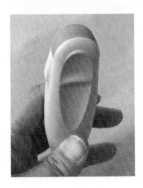

L25X 13-6 MHz linear transducer

Uses:

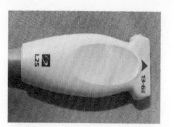

- US-guided lumbar puncture
- US-guided peripheral vascular access
- Intraosseous line confirmation
- Hip effusion/MSK
- Soft-tissue infection
- Appendix US
- Intussusception
- Pylorus US
- Ocular
- Lung pleura

Pearls:

- Lower-frequency probes are preferred over higher-frequency probes for abdominal applications in larger, older patients

PART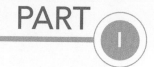

CIRCULATORY SYSTEM

1 Cardiac 3
2 Inferior vena cava 13

Cardiac

INDICATIONS

- Aid in identification of cardiac arrest during resuscitation.
- Rapidly assess the global systolic function of a patient presenting with hemodynamic instability or shock.
- Evaluate for evidence of cardiac tamponade in the setting of blunt or penetrating trauma.
- Assess patient's volume status by evaluation of inferior vena cava.
- Assess patient's response to resuscitation with serial examinations.

PROBE SELECTION

- 5-1 MHz low-frequency phased array transducer.

TECHNIQUE: (SCREEN INDICATOR LOCATED ON THE LEFT)

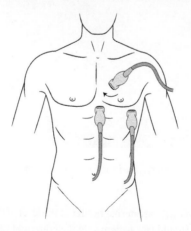

Figure 1.1 Probe placement for focused cardiac ultrasound.

Parasternal short-axis view

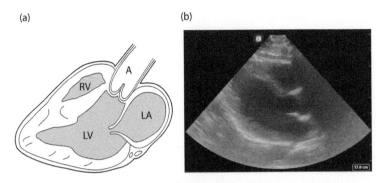

Figure 1.2 Anatomical drawing of parasternal long axis (a) with still image (b).

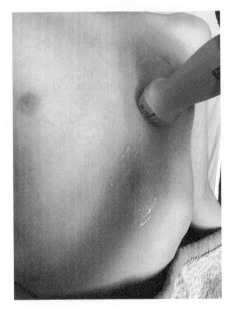

Figure 1.3 Parasternal long view. Probe indicator pointing toward the patient's left hip.

- Place probe over left parasternal border at the level of the nipple.
- Probe marker should face patient's right elbow/right hip (90° clockwise from parasternal long-axis view).

Parasternal long-axis view

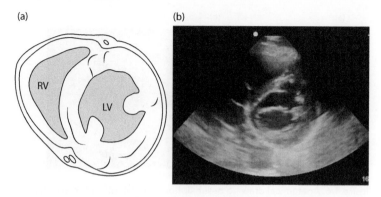

Figure 1.4 Anatomical drawing of parasternal short axis (a) with still image (b).

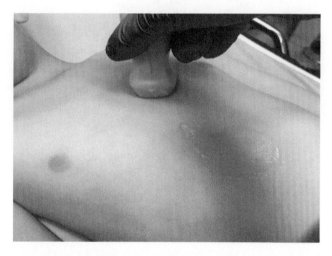

Figure 1.5 Parasternal short view. Probe indicator pointing toward the patient's right hip.

- Place probe over left parasternal border at the level of the nipple.
- Probe marker should face patient's left elbow/left hip.

6 Cardiac

Subxiphoid view

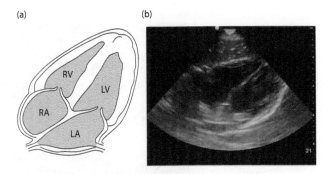

Figure 1.6 Anatomical drawing of subxiphoid view (a) with still image (b).

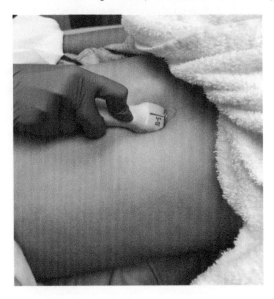

Figure 1.7 Subxiphoid view. Probe fanned from patient's right to left, using the liver as an acoustic window to visualize the heart.

- Place the probe below the xiphoid process aiming up and into the thoracic cavity.
- Use the liver as an acoustic window. Probe marker should face the patient's right.

- Apical four-chamber view
- Place probe over the point of maximal impulse (cardiac apex), generally located below the left nipple.
- Fan up and aim into the chest toward the right shoulder. (Probe marker should face the patient's right.)

Apical four-chamber view

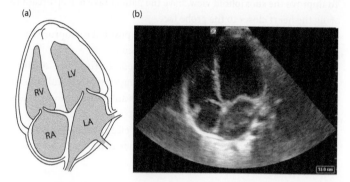

Figure 1.8 Anatomical drawing of apical four-chamber view (a) with still image (b).

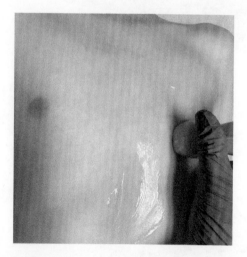

Figure 1.9 Apical four-chamber view. Probe indicator pointing toward the patient's right, usually inferior to and slightly lateral to the left nipple, with the probe face angled toward the patient's head.

- Place probe over the point of maximal impulse (cardiac apex), located below the left nipple.
- Fan up and aim into the chest toward the right shoulder. (Probe marker should face the patient's right.)

PEARLS

- To improve the subxiphoid view, have the patient take a deep breath to bring the heart closer to the probe face.
- Move the patient to the left lateral decubitus position to improve the parasternal long and apical four-chamber views.
- Differentiate a pericardial effusion from a pleural effusion by looking at the descending aorta in the parasternal long view. A pleural effusion lies behind the aorta. If the fluid collection is anterior to the aorta, it is a pericardial effusion.
- Fat pads are often mistaken with pericardial effusions. Fat pads are usually not seen in cachectic patients. Additionally, fat pads are usually only visualized anteriorly.

Parasternal long-axis view

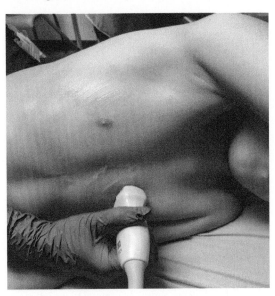

Figure 1.10 Parasternal long view in left lateral decubitus position. This allows the heart to move closer to the probe.

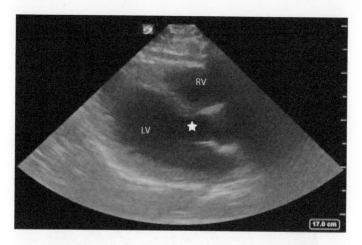

Figure 1.11 Parasternal long axis. Posterior pericardium at the bottom of the screen, with full view of the left ventricle (LV), right ventricle (RV), and aortic valve with outflow tract (star).

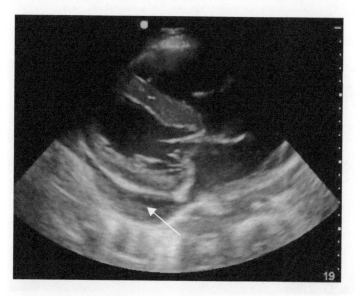

Figure 1.12 Parasternal long view of the heart with large, circumferential pericardial fluid collection (arrow).

10 Cardiac

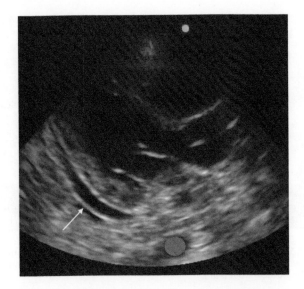

Figure 1.13 Parasternal long view of the heart with a small pericardial effusion (arrow). Notice how the fluid is located anterior to the descending aorta (red dot). This means it is a pericardial effusion (vs. a pleural effusion).

Parasternal short-axis view

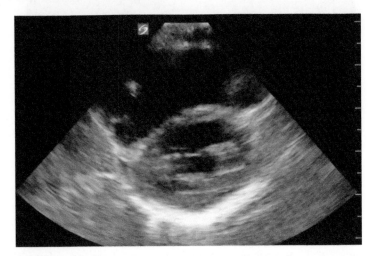

Figure 1.14 Parasternal short view with mitral valve.

Subxiphoid view

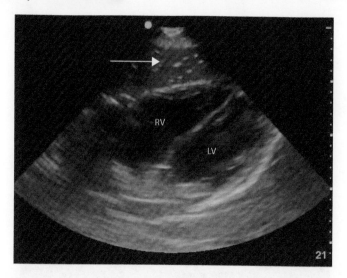

Figure 1.15 Normal subxiphoid view of the heart. The pericardium is a hyperechoic rim around the heart. The liver is a hypoechoic structure anterior to the heart (white arrow). The right ventricle (RV) and left ventricle (LV) are visible.

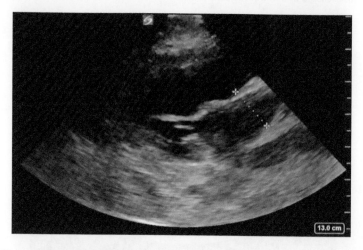

Figure 1.16 Subxiphoid view with right ventricle in nearfield and left ventricle in the farfield with chamber diameter. Notice the dilation of right ventricle compared to left.

12 Cardiac

Apical four-chamber view

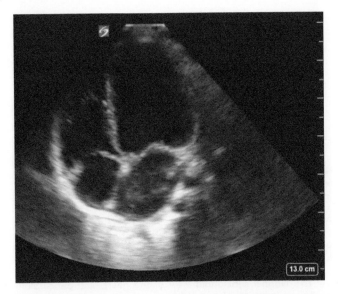

Figure 1.17 Apical four-chamber view. All four chambers of the heart visualized with tricuspid and mitral valves.

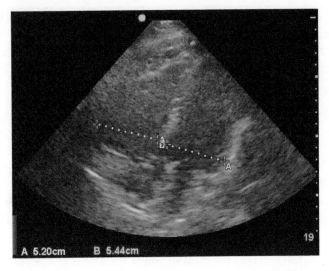

Figure 1.18 Apical four-chamber view with right ventricular dilation.

Inferior vena cava

INDICATIONS

- Assess patient's volume status.
- Assess patient's response to resuscitation with serial examinations.

PROBE SELECTION

- 5-1 MHz low-frequency phased array transducer.

TECHNIQUE

Subxiphoid view (short)

- Place transducer in the subxiphoid area with the indicator toward the patient's right.
- Identify the inferior vena cava (IVC) anterior to the spine on the patient's right, aorta on the patient's left.
- Assess the collapsibility of the IVC as the patient breathes (<50% change of IVC diameter during respiratory cycle vs. >50% change of IVC diameter, indicating the need for resuscitation).
- Measure the change in diameter approximately 2 cm distal to the right atrium insertion.

Subxiphoid view (long)

- Place the transducer in the subxiphoid area with the indicator toward the patient's head.
- Fan toward to the right to capture the IVC entering into the right side of the heart.
- Assess the collapsibility of the IVC as the patient breathes.

14 Inferior vena cava

PEARLS

- The aorta runs parallel to the IVC and can be mistaken for the IVC. Use color Doppler to differentiate between the two if you are unsure.
- Interpretation of IVC measurements should incorporate findings from the cardiac ultrasound exam (+/− lung ultrasound exam) in addition to other clinical factors such as the use of positive airway pressure.
- IVC measurements are likely more accurate when measured over time over the course of the patient's treatment and not as static one-time measurements.

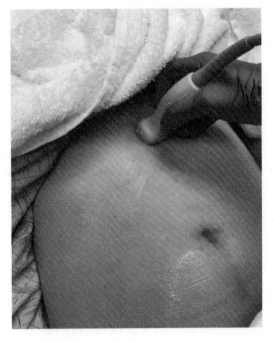

Figure 2.1 Transverse placement of the probe in the subxiphoid space.

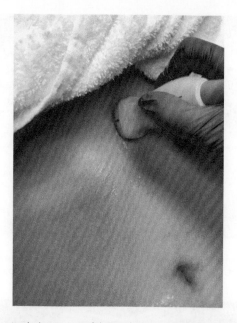

Figure 2.2 Sagittal placement of the probe in subxiphoid space.

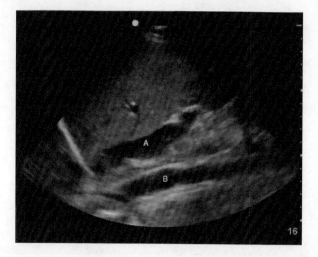

Figure 2.3 Longitudinal view of the IVC (A) and aorta (B). The IVC is proximal, adjacent to the liver with smooth hypoechoic walls. The aorta is distal to the liver with thicker, hyperechoic walls.

16 Inferior vena cava

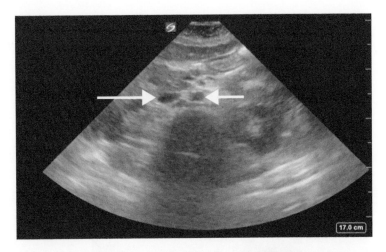

Figure 2.4 Transverse axis view of IVC (anatomical right, long arrow) and aorta (anatomical left, short arrow), with the spine and shadowing posteriorly.

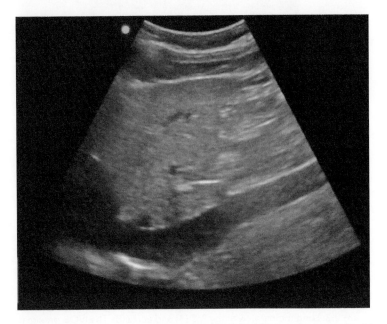

Figure 2.5 IVC entering the right atrium (lower left). IVC measurements should be taken approximately 2 cm distal to the right atrial–IVC juncture.

Pearls 17

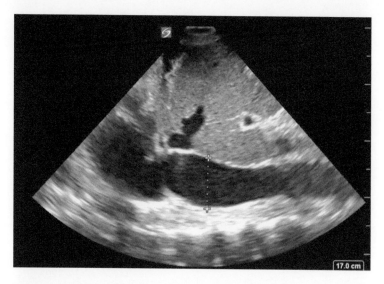

Figure 2.6 Enlarged IVC measured in the sagittal orientation.

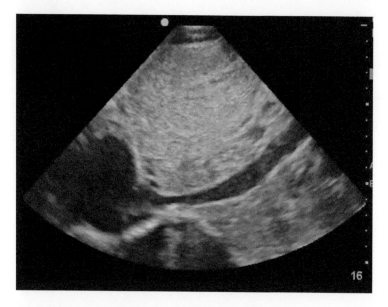

Figure 2.7 Collapse of IVC, where walls almost touch, viewed in the sagittal orientation.

PART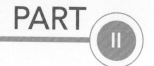

RESPIRATORY SYSTEM

3 Pulmonary   21

Pulmonary

INDICATIONS

- Evaluate lung and pleura for suspected pneumothorax, hemothorax, pleural effusion, congestive heart failure, and pneumonia.

PROBE SELECTION

- 13-6 MHz high-frequency linear transducer for pneumothorax.
- 5-2 MHz low-frequency curvilinear transducer for all other indications.

TECHNIQUE

- Place transducer in the long axis over anterior chest wall at the mid-clavicular line, and scan each interspace from cephalad to caudad.
- Look for evidence of lung sliding within each interspace along the anterior chest wall bilaterally.
- Use the same technique by using the low-frequency probe at the mid-axillary line and on the posterior thorax inferior to the scapula to thoroughly evaluate for the presence of A lines, B lines, consolidation, and pleural sliding.
- Remember to scan both diaphragms (phased array or curvilinear transducer) for hemothorax or pleural effusion by placing probe with indicator toward the patient's head, in the mid-axillary line in the right upper quadrant and the posterior axillary line in the left upper quadrant (similar to the focused assessment sonography in trauma [FAST]).

NOTES

- Pleural effusion
  - Anechoic or hypoechoic fluid collection separate from the lung above the diaphragm.

- Internal echoes within the fluid suggest the presence of hemothorax or exudate.
- A lines
  - Repetitive, horizontal artifact found in normal, dry lung.
- B lines
  - Hyperechoic, vertical lines that arise from the pleural.
  - B lines may indicate the presence of extravascular fluid or pleural disease.
- Consolidation
  - A solid appearing wedge-shaped area of the lung that appears uniformly hypoechoic.
- Pleural sliding
  - Movement of the visceral pleura against parietal pleura with the respiratory cycle.

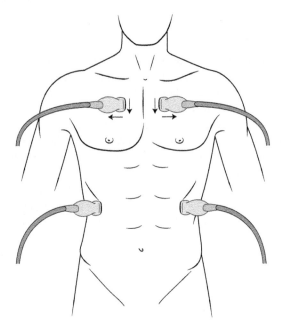

Figure 3.1 Transducer placement: Bilateral anterior chest at mid-clavicular line, bilateral chest at mid-axillary line and bilateral posterior chest at mid-clavicular line.

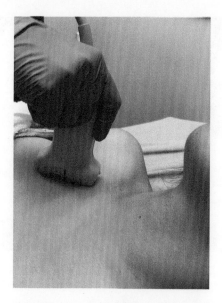

Figure 3.2 Transducer placed in the right anterior mid-clavicular line.

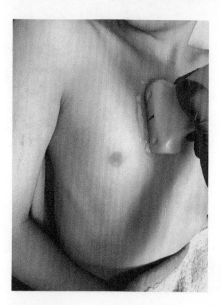

Figure 3.3 Transducer placed in the sagittal orientation on the right anterior, mid-clavicular line.

24 Pulmonary

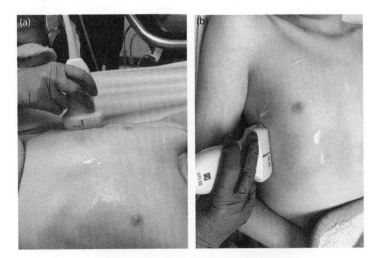

Figure 3.4 (a) Transducer placed in the sagittal orientation in the mid-axillary line. (b) Transducer placed in the sagittal orientation in the mid-axillary line.

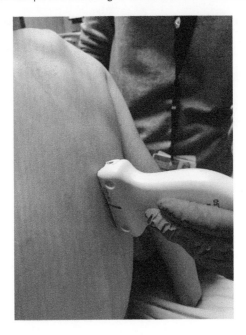

Figure 3.5 Transducer in the sagittal orientation inferior to the scapula.

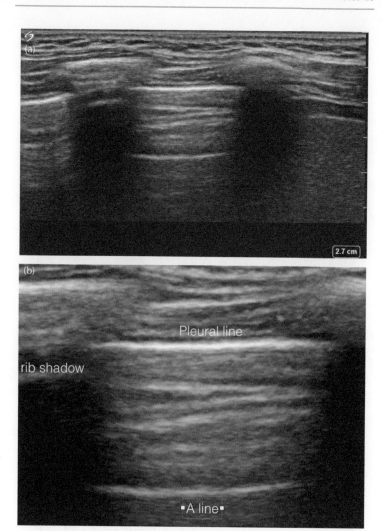

Figure 3.6 (a) Normal lung in the sagittal probe orientation. Pleural line between rib shadows with A line beneath. (b) Zoomed in appearance of normal aerated lung in the sagittal orientation showing rib shadowing, pleural line with A lines present.

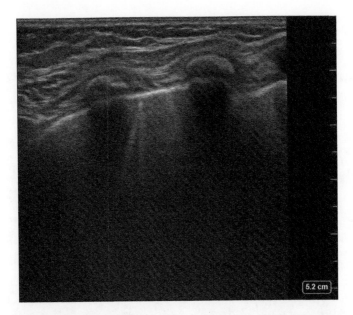

Figure 3.7 B lines in the sagittal probe orientation. Vertical echogenic lines originating from the pleura.

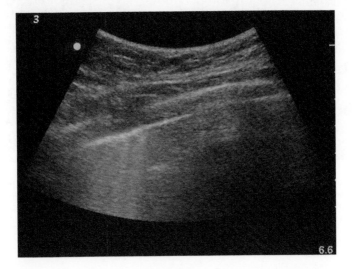

Figure 3.8 Multiple B lines originating from the pleura.

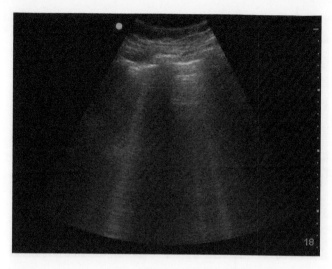

Figure 3.9 Multiple B lines within an intercostal space. More than three B lines within an intercostal space are indicative of extravascular lung water in the appropriate clinical setting.

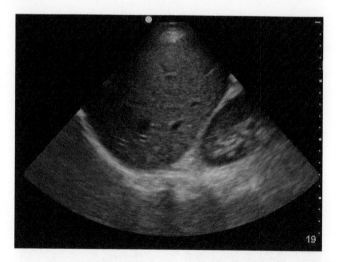

Figure 3.10 Right upper quadrant (RUQ) view. Thoracic spine (scalloped hyperechoic line at bottom of screen) meets diaphragm (hyperechoic stripe superior to the liver). The lung is normal and aerated. The spine does not continue past the diaphragm.

28 Pulmonary

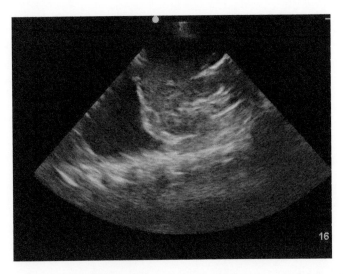

Figure 3.11 RUQ view showing "spine sign." The spine continues past the diaphragm due to the presence of a pleural effusion.

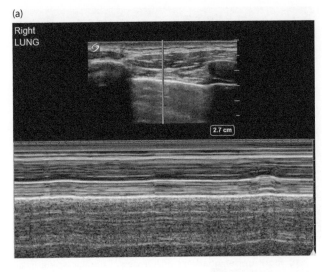

Figure 3.12 (a) Normal lung. Pleural sliding present in M mode. (*Continued*)

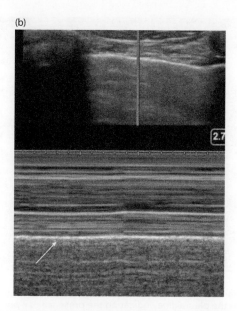

Figure 3.12 (*Continued*) (b) Zoomed still image of (a) with pleura (arrow). Place M mode cursor on the pleura. The screen should show no movement separated by a hyperechoic line (arrow) with movement below the pleura.

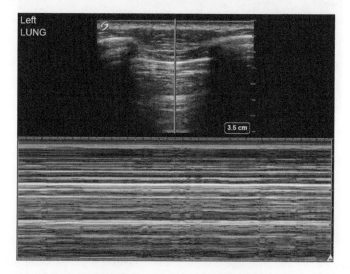

Figure 3.13 Pneumothorax.

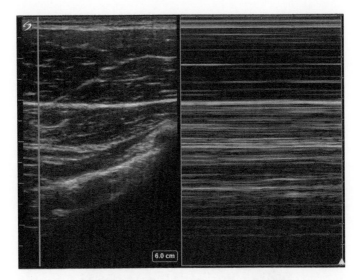

Figure 3.14 Evaluation of abnormal pleura using M mode. No sign of movement above or below the pleural line, indicating the presence of a pneumothorax.

(a)

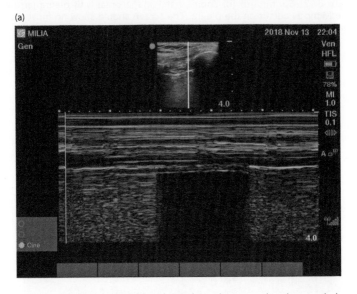

Figure 3.15 Lung point sign. The place where the visceral and parietal pleura begins to separate in the presence of a pneumothorax, which is caught on ultrasound. *(Continued)*

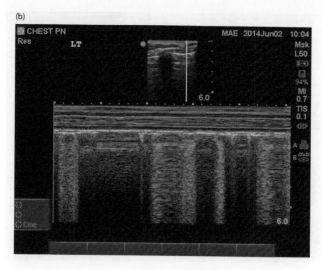

Figure 3.15 (*Continued*) Lung point sign. The place where the visceral and parietal pleura begins to separate in the presence of a pneumothorax, which is caught on ultrasound.

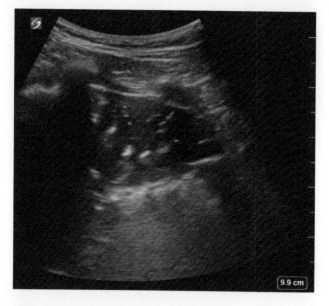

Figure 3.16 Pneumonia in consolidated lung can appear with white specks (air bronchograms) that move up and down with the respiratory cycle.

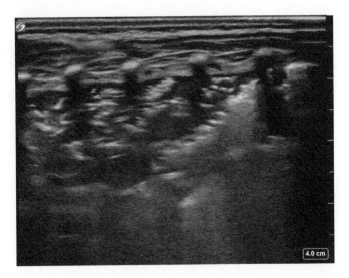

Figure 3.17 Sagittal view of pneumonia with air bronchograms.

PART III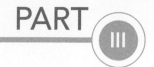

MUSCULOSKELETAL SYSTEM

4	Long bone	35
5	Clavicle	43
6	Shoulder	49
7	Elbow	53
8	Hip	61
9	Knee	67
10	Ankle	75

4

Long bone

INDICATIONS

- Assess patients with history or exam concerning a long bone fracture.

PROBE SELECTION

- 13-6 MHz high-frequency linear transducer.

TECHNIQUE

- Scan in two planes (both longitudinal and transverse) over the bone looking for a disruption of the cortex.
- Bony cortex will look like a hyperechoic line with posterior shadowing.
- Muscle fibers have a spindle-like appearance in longitudinal scans and a speckled appearance in transverse scans.
- Scan the unaffected side for comparison.

PEARLS

- In the sagittal plane, place the probe directly over the bone at 90° so that you can see the entirety of the shaft.
- Growth plates and fractures can be mistaken for one another and thus it may be helpful to scan the unaffected side for comparison. Ultrasound for long bone fractures should be used in conjunction with radiography for high risk or high mechanism patients.

36 Long bone

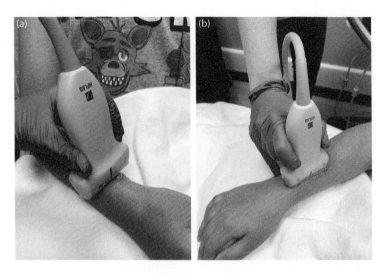

Figure 4.1 (a) Distal radius in the transverse orientation. (b) Distal radius in the sagittal orientation.

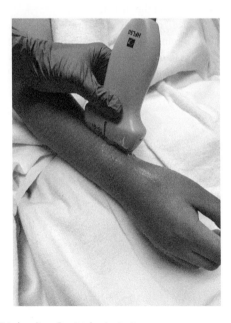

Figure 4.2 Distal radius. Sagittal orientation.

Pearls 37

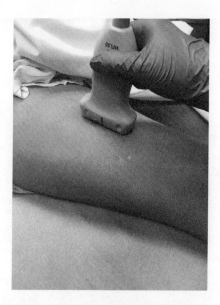

Figure 4.3 Femur bone. Sagittal orientation.

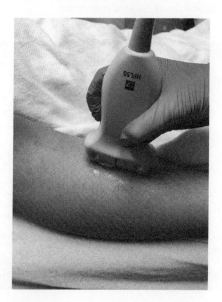

Figure 4.4 Tibia bone. Sagittal orientation.

38 Long bone

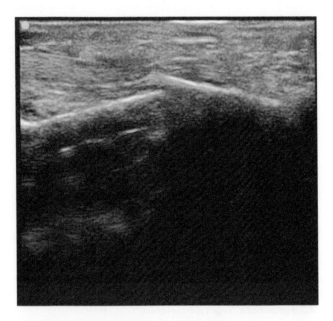

Figure 4.5 Displaced fracture. Sagittal orientation.

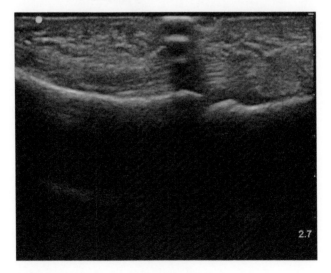

Figure 4.6 Displaced fracture. Sagittal orientation.

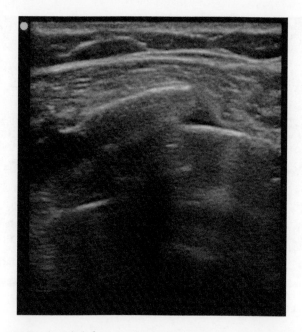

Figure 4.7 Displaced rib fracture. Sagittal orientation.

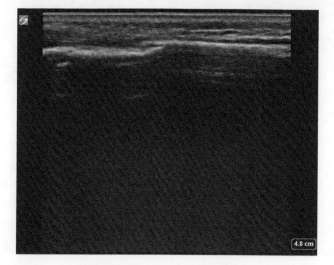

Figure 4.8 Fracture of the tibia in sagittal orientation.

40 Long bone

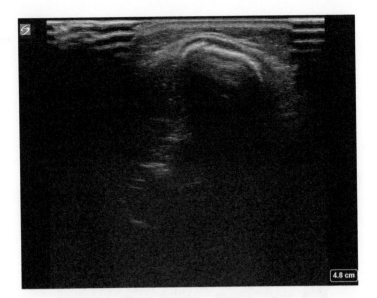

Figure 4.9 Fracture of tibia in transverse orientation.

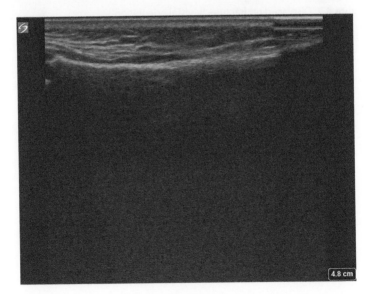

Figure 4.10 Normal tibia bone in sagittal orientation.

Pearls 41

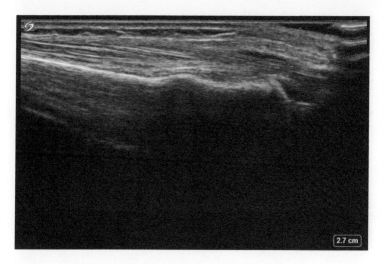

Figure 4.11 Buckle fracture of radius in sagittal orientation.

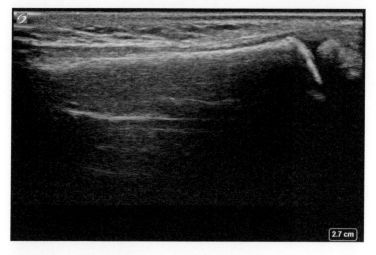

Figure 4.12 Normal radius bone in sagittal orientation.

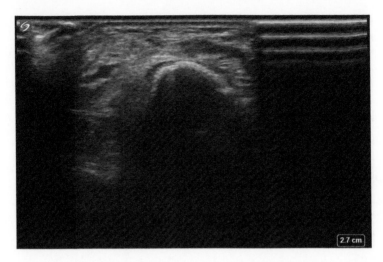

Figure 4.13 Buckle fracture of radius in transverse orientation.

5

Clavicle

INDICATIONS

- Assess patients with history or exam concerning for a clavicle fracture.

PROBE SELECTION

- High-frequency linear transducer or low-frequency curvilinear transducer.

TECHNIQUE

- Scan in two planes (both longitudinal and transverse) directly over the clavicle bone, looking for a disruption of the cortex.
- The bone will appear as a hyperechoic structure with posterior shadowing.
- A hematoma may be visualized in an acute fracture, which will appear as anechoic fluid adjacent to the fracture.
- Scan the unaffected side for comparison.

PEARLS

- Compare the affected side with the unaffected side to ensure that an abnormality exists.

44 Clavicle

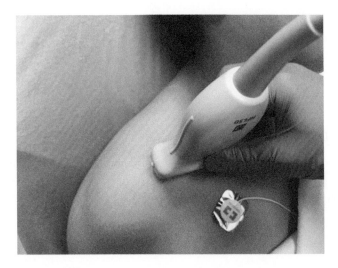

Figure 5.1 Longitudinal orientation with probe placed in supra-clavicular notch.

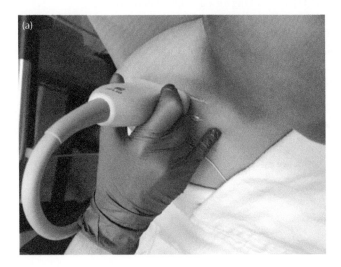

Figure 5.2 (a,b) Longitudinal orientation with probe placed directly on the clavicle. (*Continued*)

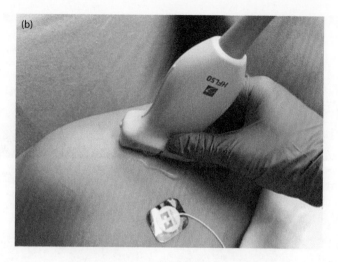

Figure 5.2 (*Continued*) (a,b) Longitudinal orientation with probe placed directly on the clavicle.

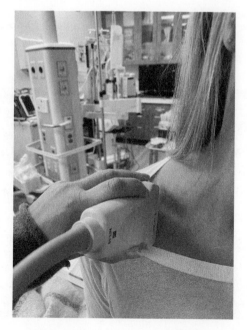

Figure 5.3 Probe placed in transverse orientation over the clavicle.

46 Clavicle

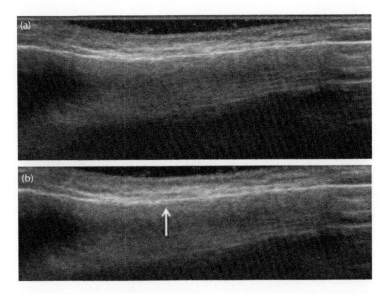

Figure 5.4 Normal clavicle in the longitudinal orientation (a). Clavicle is a hyperechoic line (white arrow), which continues the line across the upper screen (b).

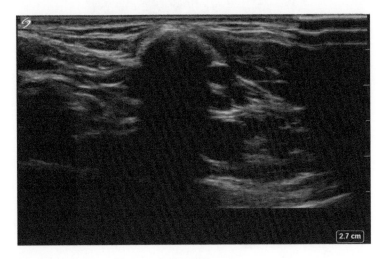

Figure 5.5 Normal clavicle in the transverse axis.

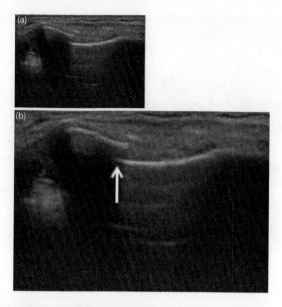

Figure 5.6 Fracture of the clavicle in the longitudinal orientation (a). Fracture appears as a disruption of the cortex (b).

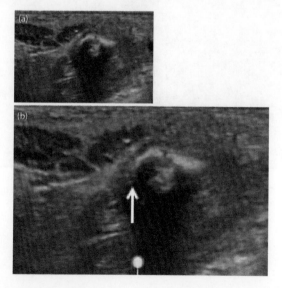

Figure 5.7 Fracture of the clavicle in the transverse orientation (a). Note disruption (white arrow) in the cortex (b).

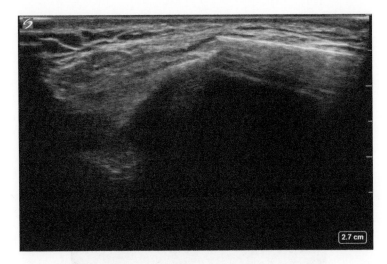

Figure 5.8 Sagittal view of clavicle fracture.

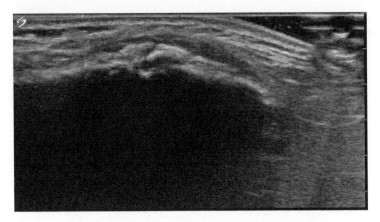

Figure 5.9 Sagittal view of old clavicle fracture. Bone thickening and incomplete union present.

6

Shoulder

INDICATIONS

- Assess the joint for effusion, dislocation, tendon injury.
- Reassessment after joint reduction.
- Ultrasound guidance for regional anesthesia or joint aspiration.

PROBE SELECTION

- High-frequency linear transducer or low-frequency curvilinear transducer.

TECHNIQUE

Posterior view

- The patient should be seated with the back toward the sonographer with ultrasound machine to the side or in front of the patient within the sonographer's view.
- Place the probe on posterior shoulder at the level of the scapular spine parallel to the floor with the probe marker facing to the patients left.
- Scan antero-laterally until the glenohumeral joint is visualized.

PEARLS

- Use the posterior view if an anterior shoulder dislocation is suspected.
- If the shoulder anatomy is difficult to visualize, internally and externally rotate the shoulder with the ultrasound to better demonstrate the relationship of the humeral head and glenoid.

50 Shoulder

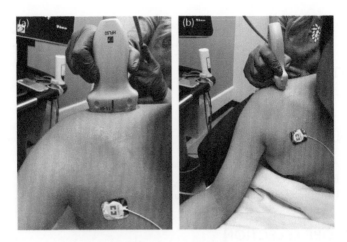

Figure 6.1 (a) Start with probe placed directly over the top of the shoulder. (b) Slide probe toward the clavicle until it is directly over the acromioclavicular joint.

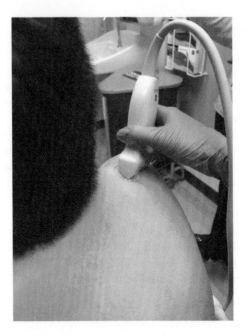

Figure 6.2 Start with probe at the level of the scapular spine parallel to the floor. Scan anterolaterally until the glenohumeral joint is visualized.

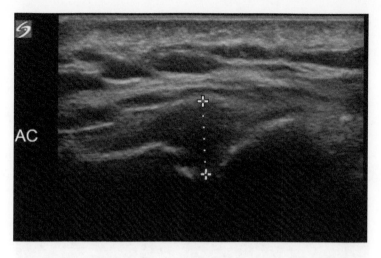

Figure 6.3 Shoulder joint effusion (hypoechoic fluid collection between two white crosses).

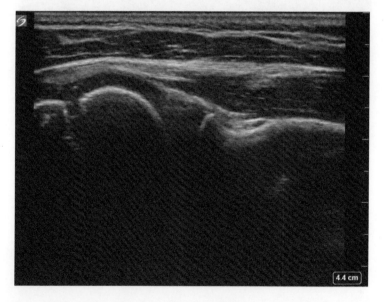

Figure 6.4 Posterior view of the shoulder at the glenohumeral joint.

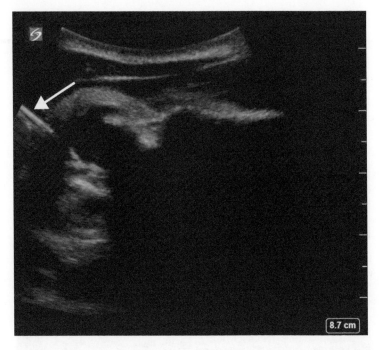

Figure 6.5 Hematoma block for regional anesthesia; note the hyperechoic needle from the left side of the screen being inserted directly into the hematoma at the glenohumeral joint.

7

Elbow

INDICATIONS

- Assess for joint effusion, fracture, tendon, or ligamentous injury.

PROBE SELECTION

- High-frequency linear transducer or low-frequency curvilinear transducer.

TECHNIQUE

Anterior view

- Place the probe on the anterior aspect of the distal humerus with the patient's elbow in extension.
- Scan in the longitudinal plane moving cephalad from the distal humerus and in the transverse plane at the coronoid fossa.

Posterior view

- Place the elbow in 90° of flexion with probe on the posterior aspect of the distal humerus.
- Scan in both the longitudinal and transverse axes.

PEARLS

- Compare findings to those of the unaffected joint.
- Posterior approach to the elbow is preferred for arthrocentesis.
- Always look for the "triangle" in the elbow, made of the lateral epicondyle of the humerus, the radial head, and the olecranon.

54 Elbow

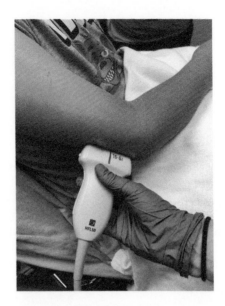

Figure 7.1 Posterior sagittal approach.

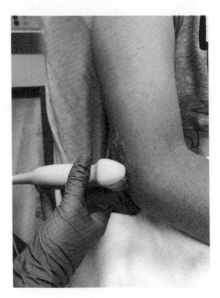

Figure 7.2 Posterior transverse approach.

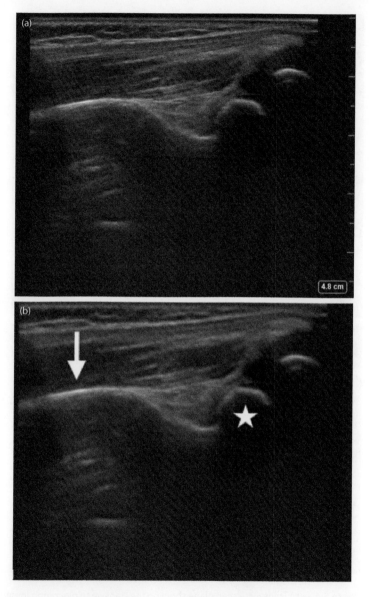

Figure 7.3 (a,b) Normal elbow in the sagittal orientation. Radial head (star) and lateral epicondyle (arrow). The extensor tendon lies above these structures near the surface.

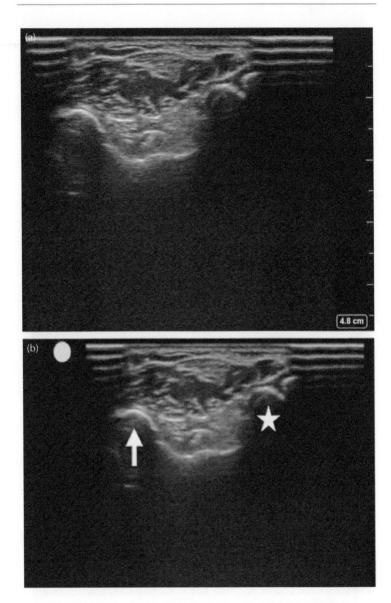

Figure 7.4 (a,b) Transverse scan plane showing the transverse olecranon fossa between the radius and ulna (star and arrow).

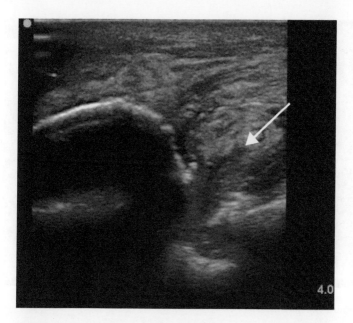

Figure 7.5 Elbow joint effusion (white arrow).

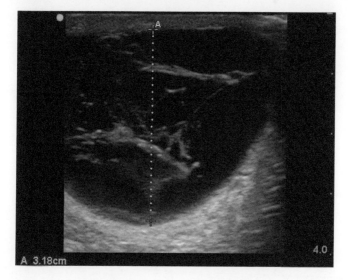

Figure 7.6 Bursitis. Bursal sac filled with hypoechoic fluid with internal echoes.

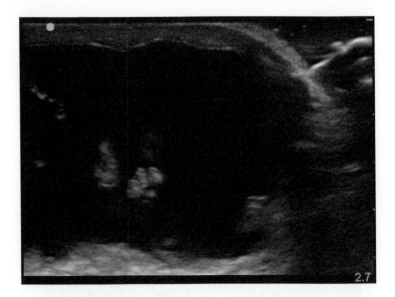

Figure 7.7 Bursitis.

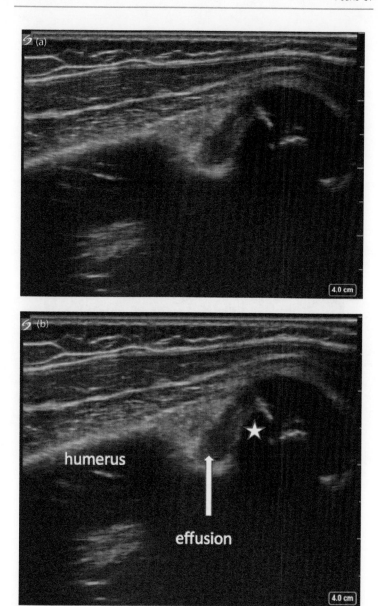

Figure 7.8 Elbow effusion in the sagittal orientation. Humerus, olecranon (star) and effusion.

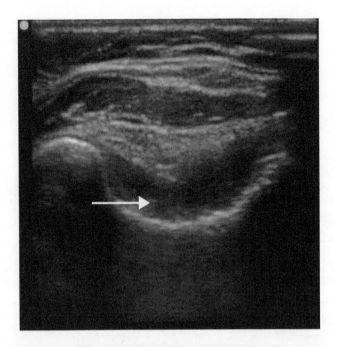

Figure 7.9 Elbow effusion (white arrow) in transverse orientation.

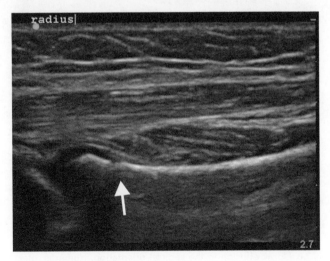

Figure 7.10 Elbow fracture (white arrow) with overlying effusion.

Hip

INDICATIONS

- Assess the hip joint for the presence of effusion.
- Assess patients who present with a limp, refusal to bear weight, or painful extremity or hip.

PROBE SELECTION

- High-frequency linear transducer or low-frequency curvilinear transducer.

TECHNIQUE

- Place legs in a neutral position with hip slightly externally rotated.
- Place the transducer parallel to the long axis of the femoral neck.
- Measure from the anterior concavity of the femoral neck to the posterior surface of the iliopsoas muscle.

PEARLS

- Perform the ultrasound on the unaffected side for comparison.
- An effusion is defined as anterior synovial space thickness >5 mm or >2 mm difference when compared to asymptomatic side.

62 Hip

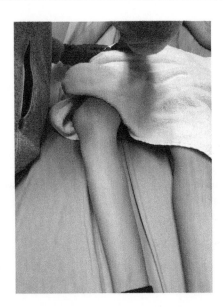

Figure 8.1 Lying in a supine position, gently externally rotate the hip with the knee flexed.

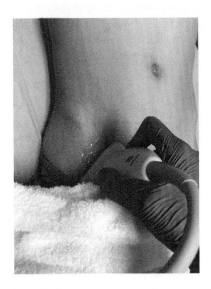

Figure 8.2 Probe in sagittal plane.

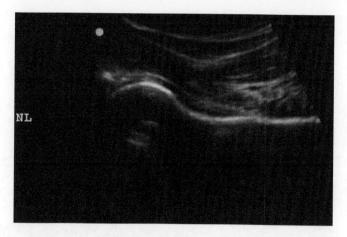

Figure 8.3 Normal hip. Sagittal view

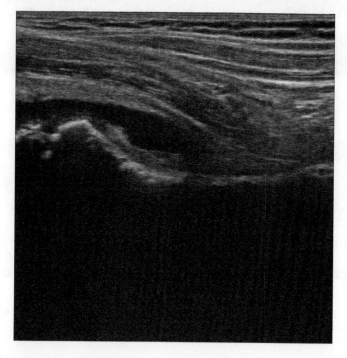

Figure 8.4 Normal hip. Sagittal orientation. A normal amount of joint fluid is present. An effusion is significant only if it is >5 mm in thickness.

64 Hip

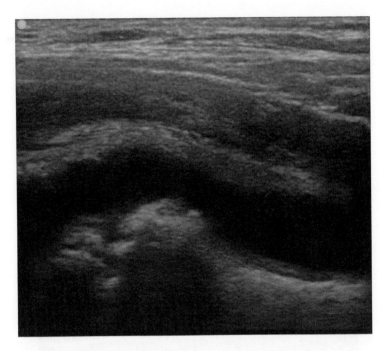

Figure 8.5 Hip effusion. Fluid collection is >5 mm in thickness.

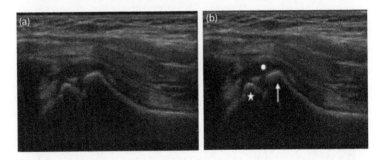

Figure 8.6 In-plane evaluation of the hip joint in the longitudinal orientation (a). (b) Shows the femoral capital epiphysis (star), femoral metaphysics (arrow), and anterior synovial space (circle).

Pearls 65

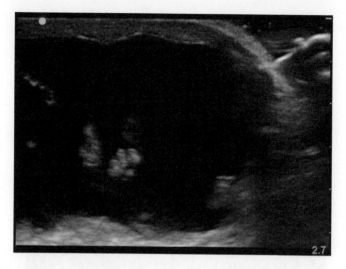

Figure 8.7 Hip joint effusion. Sagittal orientation showing a significant fluid collection >5 mm in diameter.

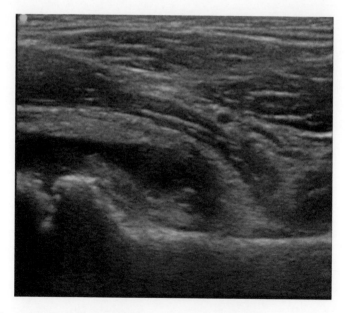

Figure 8.8 Sagittal view of the hip with a large joint effusion.

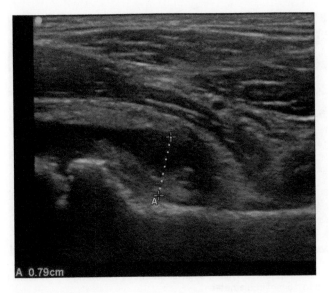

Figure 8.9 Hip effusion.

9

Knee

INDICATIONS

- Evaluate for knee effusion; hemarthrosis; tendon, ligamentous, or muscular injuries; or fractures.
- Ultrasound guidance for joint injections or aspirations.

PROBE SELECTION

- High-frequency linear transducer.

TECHNIQUE

- Place the patient in the supine position with the knee in flexion.
- Place the probe in the midline of the knee anteriorly in the sagittal plane just superior to the patella and scan caudad to where the quadriceps tendon inserts into the patella; rotate the probe 90° to obtain view in transverse orientation.
- Continue inferiorly and obtain a sagittal view of the patellar tendon at its insertion point at the tibial tuberosity. Rotate the probe 90° to obtain a transverse view.
- Evaluate the medial and lateral collateral ligaments in the sagittal orientation.

PEARLS

- Open physes can be mistaken for fractures.
- Compare the affected side with the unaffected side to ensure that an abnormality exists.

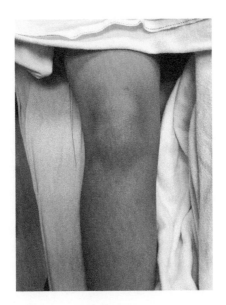

Figure 9.1 Normal anterior view of a knee.

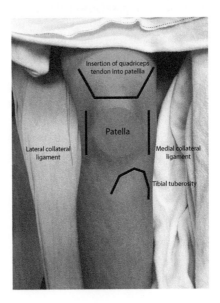

Figure 9.2 Major anatomical features of the knee.

Pearls 69

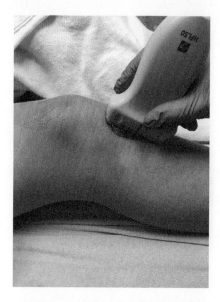

Figure 9.3 Anterior longitudinal probe placement. Infrapatellar.

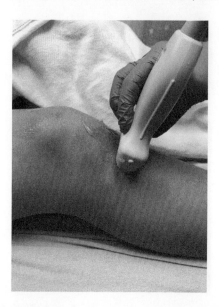

Figure 9.4 Anterior transverse probe placement. Lateral condyles.

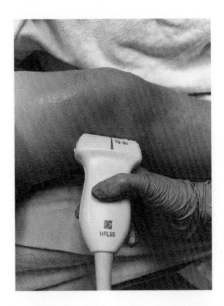

Figure 9.5 Anterior longitudinal probe placement. Lateral collateral ligament.

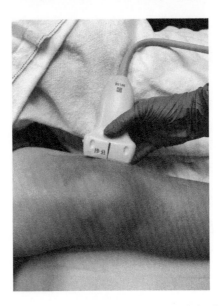

Figure 9.6 Anterior longitudinal probe placement. Medial collateral ligament.

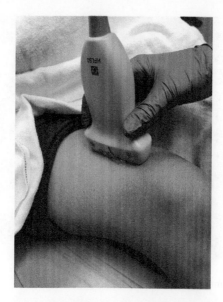

Figure 9.7 Anterior longitudinal probe placement. Suprapatellar.

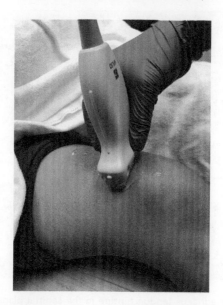

Figure 9.8 Anterior transverse probe placement.

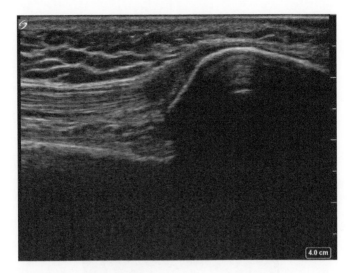

Figure 9.9 Normal knee.

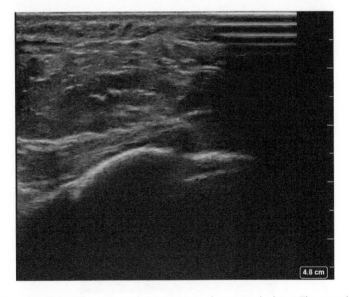

Figure 9.10 Quadriceps tendon rupture in the sagittal plane. The muscle tendon layers are disrupted.

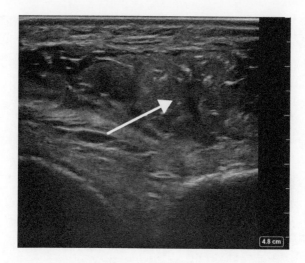

Figure 9.11 Quadriceps tendon rupture with hematoma (white arrow).

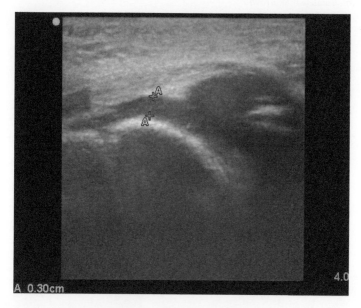

Figure 9.12 Prepatellar septic bursitis. The bursa contains hypoechoic fluid with internal echoes. The subcutaneous tissues above the bursa are inflamed.

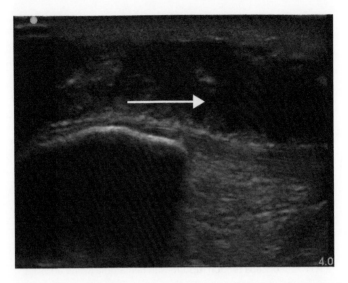

Figure 9.13 Prepatellar bursitis. Sagittal plane showing a large fluid collection in the bursa (white arrow).

Ankle

INDICATIONS

- Assess for joint effusion, tendon or ligamentous injury, or fracture.
- Ultrasound guidance for joint aspiration or regional anesthesia.

PROBE SELECTION

- High-frequency linear transducer.

TECHNIQUE

Anterior view

- Place the patient in the supine position with the foot in slight dorsiflexion.
- Place the probe on the distal tibia in the longitudinal axis sliding inferiorly until the tibia, joint space, and talus are visualized. Turn the probe 90° to obtain the transverse view.

Posterior view

- Have the patient lay prone with the foot hanging off the side of the bed.
- Place the probe in the longitudinal axis along the Achilles tendon at its point of insertion on the calcaneus.
- Turn the probe 90° to obtain the transverse view.

PEARLS

- Ankle effusions are best viewed from an anterior approach.
- Compare the affected side with the unaffected side to ensure an abnormality exists.

76 Ankle

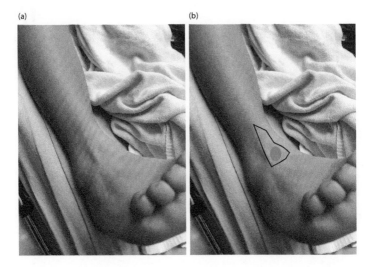

Figure 10.1 (a) View of anterior ankle. (b) Ankle triangle. Lateral: Extensor digitorum longus; medial anterior tibilias. Blue dot: Dorsalis pedis artery.

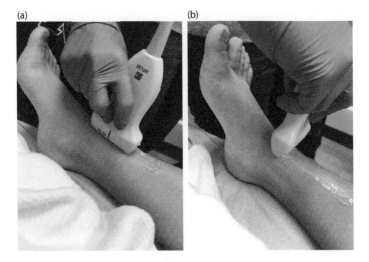

Figure 10.2 (a) Anterior placement of probe in the sagittal plane. (b) Anterior placement of probe in the transverse plane.

Pearls 77

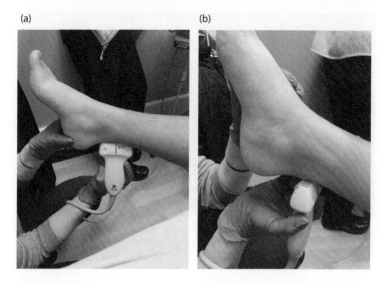

Figure 10.3 (a) Posterior placement of probe in sagittal plane. (b) Posterior placement of probe in transverse plane.

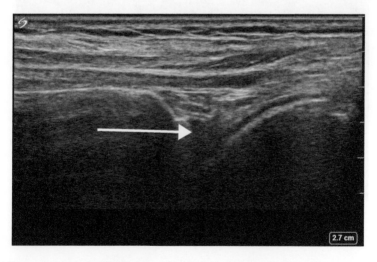

Figure 10.4 Normal ankle. Sagittal orientation. Joint space (arrow).

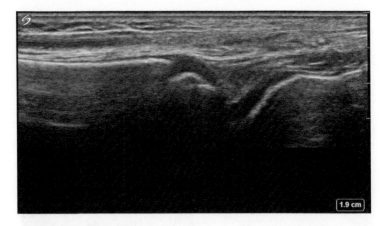

Figure 10.5 Ankle effusion.

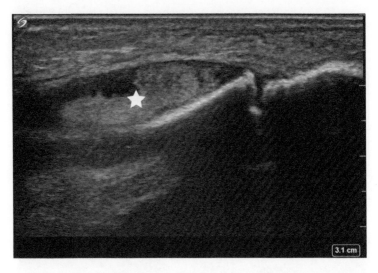

Figure 10.6 Anterior sagittal view with abscess (*) overlying distal tibia.

Pearls 79

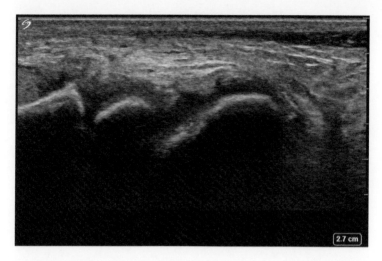

Figure 10.7 Sagittal view of tibiotalar joint with small effusion and irregular appearance of muscle overlying effusion.

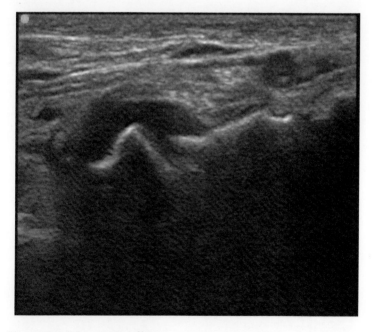

Figure 10.8 Talonavicular effusion.

PART IV

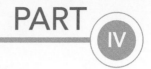

INTEGUMENTARY SYSTEM

| 11 Soft-tissue | 83 |
| 12 Neck | 93 |

PART

Soft-tissue

INDICATIONS

- Assess soft-tissue masses, foreign bodies, fluid collections, swelling, infection.

PROBE SELECTION

- High-frequency linear transducer.

TECHNIQUE

- Most soft-tissue findings are located superficially. Minimize depth to improve visualization.
- Place probe in the center of area of interest in the sagittal orientation. Slowly scan left to right across entirety of soft-tissue finding. Rotate probe 90° and scan the soft-tissue finding in the transverse orientation moving the probe cephalad to caudad.
- If accurate measurements of the soft-tissue finding are important, slide the probe across the skin surface. Do not fan.
- Take note of the location, depth, surrounding vascular or nerve structures.
- Place color Doppler on the soft-tissue finding to determine if there is vascular flow.

PEARLS

- Scan in two planes to understand the true size of the soft-tissue finding.
- Use color Doppler to determine if there is vascular flow.
- Note the depth and surrounding structures of the soft-tissue finding. If it is very deep or surrounded by delicate structures such as nerves or blood vessels, a simple extraction or incision and drainage may not be appropriate.

- Foreign body
  - Radio-opaque and radiolucent foreign bodies appear hyperechoic on ultrasound.
  - Posterior acoustic shadowing allows the foreign body to be easily detected within the skin and soft tissue.
- Cellulitis
  - Inflammation and edema causes soft tissue to have a "smudged" appearance. However, the fascial planes remain intact.
  - In later stages, soft tissue has a lobular appearance, often coined as "cobblestones."
  - Any edema will cause appearance of cobblestoning so clinical correlation is necessary to determine if this is cellulitis or edema from another cause.
- Abscess
  - Hypoechoic fluid collection with irregular borders and internal echoes, with posterior acoustic enhancement, surrounded by the inflamed tissue.

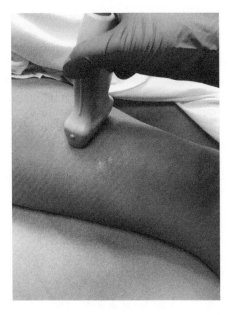

Figure 11.1 Probe placed directly over the center of soft-tissue finding. Transverse probe orientation.

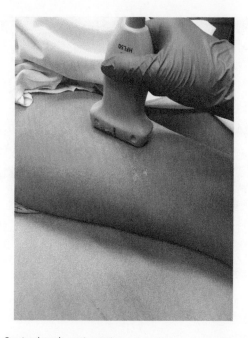

Figure 11.2 Sagittal probe orientation.

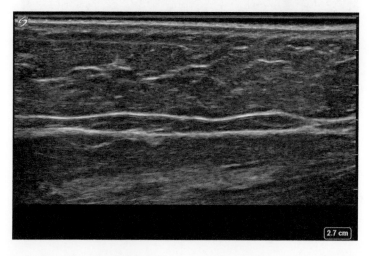

Figure 11.3 Normal soft tissue. You can see the epidermis, dermis, soft tissue and muscle layers.

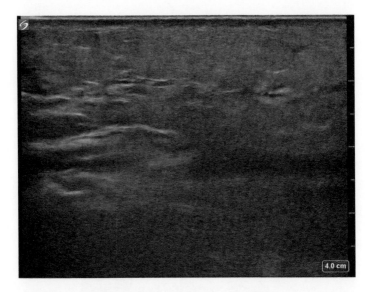

Figure 11.4 Early cellulitis. The soft tissue is hyperechoic in comparison to surrounding tissue, and may be thickened.

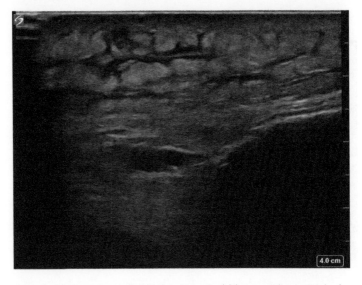

Figure 11.5 Later stage cellulitis showing a "cobblestone" (interstitial edema surrounding fat lobules).

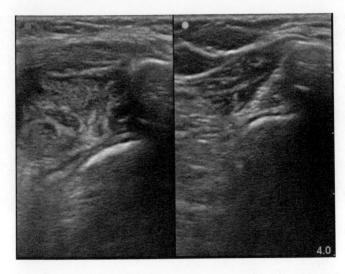

Figure 11.8 Pyomyositis. Ultrasound can distinguish between superficial abscesses and deeper infections in muscle tissue such as pyomyositis.

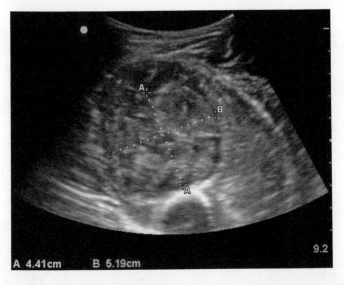

Figure 11.9 Thigh hematoma. Hematomas are usually oval to lenticular, can be well demarcated but have irregular borders, hypoechoic with internal echoes. Hematomas can be sonographically similar to abscesses, so history and exam findings can be important distinguishing factors.

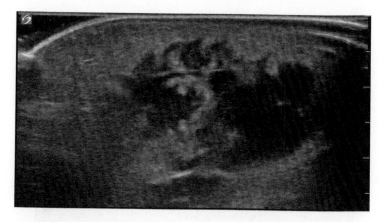

Figure 11.6 Abscess.

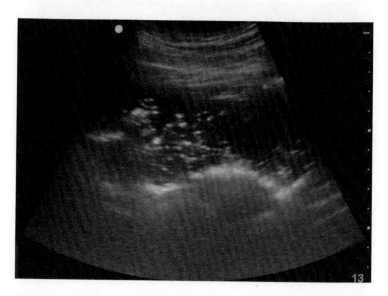

Figure 11.7 Abscess. Fluid collection with internal echoes and irregular borders.

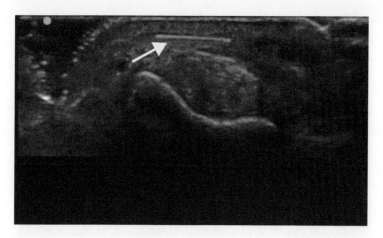

Figure 11.10 Linear foreign body (arrow).

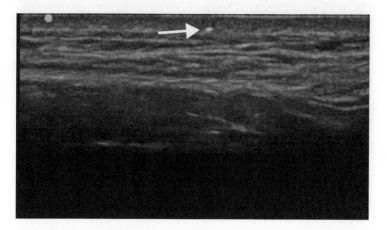

Figure 11.11 Punctate foreign body (arrow).

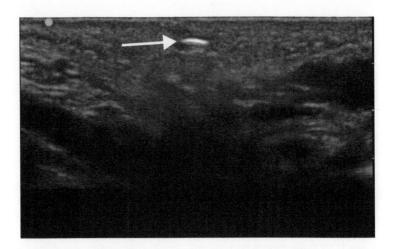

Figure 11.12 Foreign body (arrow).

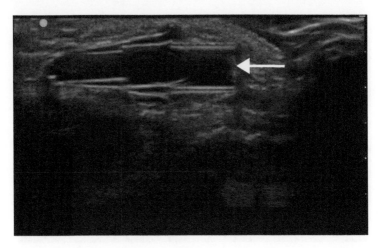

Figure 11.13 Hollow foreign body (arrow).

Pearls 91

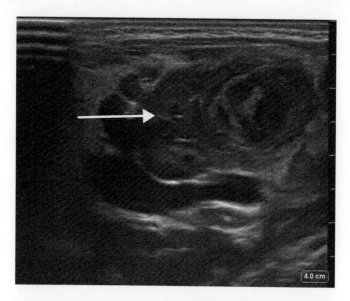

Figure 11.14 Abscess adjacent to a blood vessel (arrow).

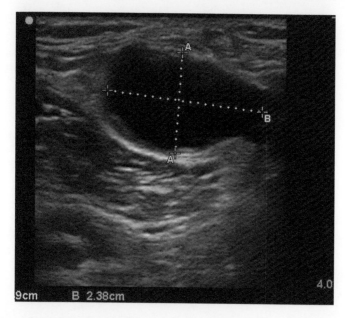

Figure 11.15 Baker's cyst. Cysts are usually ovoid, well demarcated with thin walls, without surrounding inflammatory soft-tissue changes.

12

Neck

INDICATIONS

- Evaluate neck masses and pre-procedure evaluation of neck vasculature.

PROBE SELECTION

- High-frequency linear transducer.

TECHNIQUE

- Place the patient in the supine position with the neck in hyperextension. If the area of evaluation is on one side of the face or neck, turn the patient's head to the side to optimize positioning.
- Scan through the entire area of interest in both transverse and sagittal planes.

PEARLS

- Obtain images of the contralateral side of the neck to obtain comparison views.
- Use color flow imaging to distinguish vasculature from fluid-filled masses or nerves.

94 Neck

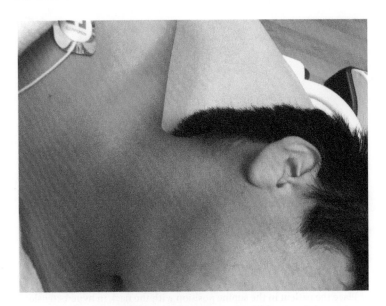

Figure 12.1 Patient positioning: Hyperextension and flexion of the neck.

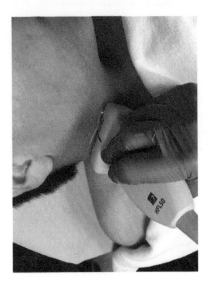

Figure 12.2 Placement of probe in transverse orientation to maximize probe surface area.

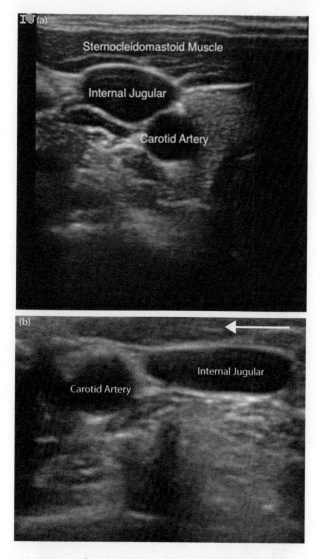

Figure 12.3 Views of arterial and venous vasculature in lateral neck in transverse orientation. The internal jugular vein is often located either anterior to (a) or adjacent to (b) the carotid artery. The internal jugular vein is often easily compressible, ovoid in shape, lying just beneath the sternocleidomastoid muscle (white arrow). The carotid artery is more circular, located either posterior to or adjacent to the internal jugular vein.

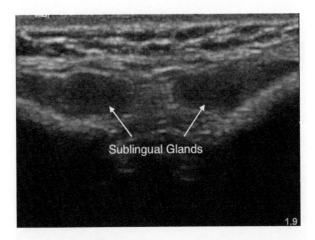

Figure 12.4 Sublingual glands are very small, and sometimes can only be seen if there is pathology. Placement of the probe in the transverse orientation under the chin (submental) can produce the image above.

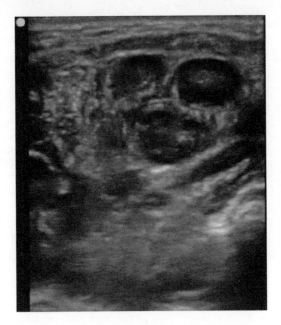

Figure 12.5 Lymph nodes. Benign lymph nodes often have an elliptical shape, with an echogenic hilus and preserved sinusoidal architecture.

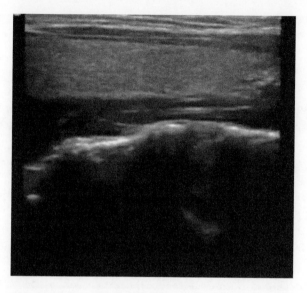

Figure 12.6 Sagittal view of the thyroid and the trachea along the lateral aspect of the neck. This view can be obtained by placing the probe just lateral to the laryngeal prominence.

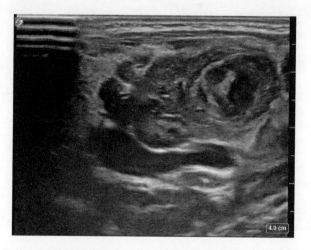

Figure 12.7 Sagittal view of a fluctuant mass (abscess) on the neck, just lateral to a blood vessel. Abscesses often have irregular, poorly defined borders, containing fluid with varying echogenicities. Absence of color Doppler flow differentiates abscesses from lymph nodes, other growths, or malignancies.

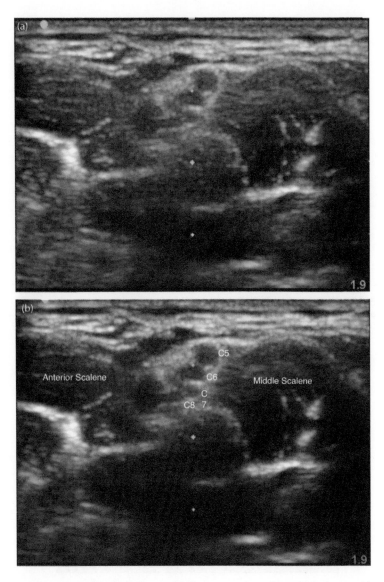

Figure 12.8 (a) Brachial plexus. (b) Short-axis view of brachial plexus with anatomical landmarks.

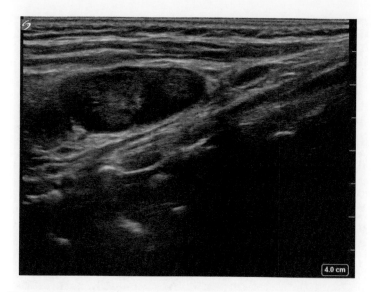

Figure 12.9 Lymph node.

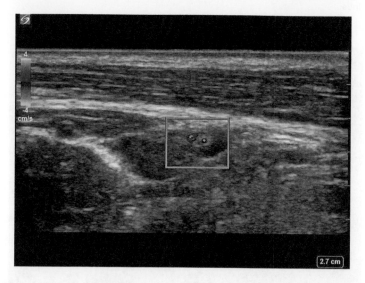

Figure 12.10 Small lymph node in anterior cervical chain with flow in the sinus.

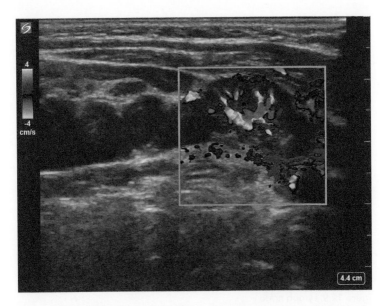

Figure 12.11 Enlarged lymph node in amterior cervical chain with flow in the sinus.

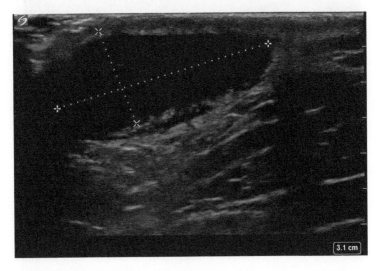

Figure 12.12 Cyst in neck.

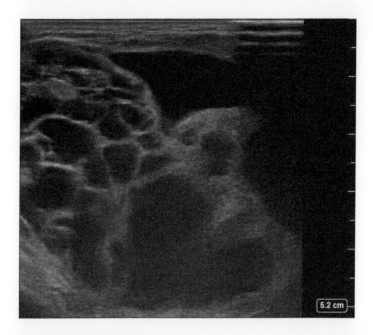

Figure 12.13 Cystic hygroma.

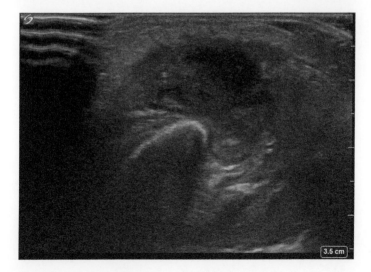

Figure 12.14 Submandibular gland abscess.

PART V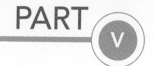

DIGESTIVE SYSTEM

13	Appendix	105
14	Intussusception	111
15	Pylorus	117
16	Biliary	121

Appendix

INDICATIONS

- Assess patients with a history or physical exam concerning for acute appendicitis.

PROBE SELECTION

- High-frequency linear transducer (may need to use curvilinear transducer in patients with large BMI).

TECHNIQUE

- Use the graded compression technique.*
- Localize the source of pain.
- Place the probe on the point of maximal tenderness, marker to the patient's right.
- Evaluate area in both the short and long axis.
- Look for a rounded, non-compressible tube-like structure with a diameter greater than 6 mm.

PEARLS

- Measure the appendix from the outer wall to outer wall.
- Evaluate for secondary signs of inflammation such as peri-appendiceal inflammation, free fluid, or an appendicolith.

---

* Graded compression is the technique of moving the abdominal probe in the area of concern with episodes of gentle compression on the skin surface. The goal is to displace or move anatomical structures to improve visualization. This technique is commonly used to evaluate the appendix.

- Note the presence of hyperemia in the appendiceal wall (which can be appreciated by placing color Doppler on the wall of the appendix), often termed the "ring of fire."

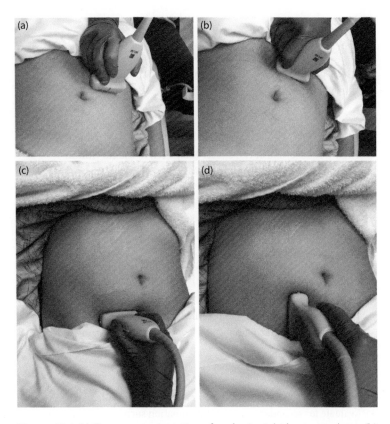

Figure 13.1 (a) Transverse orientation of probe in right lower quadrant. (b) Graded compression with the probe in transverse orientation, moving caudad (a) to cephalad. (c) Continued movement of probe caudad; then moving the probe horizontally and moving cephalad again (lawnmower technique). (d) Rotate probe 90° and repeat in the sagittal orientation, moving horizontally from left to right and then vertically.

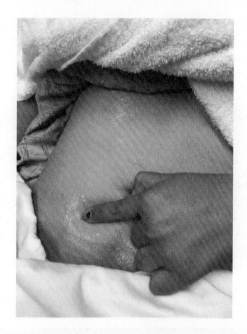

Figure 13.2 Having patient point to maximal area of tenderness.

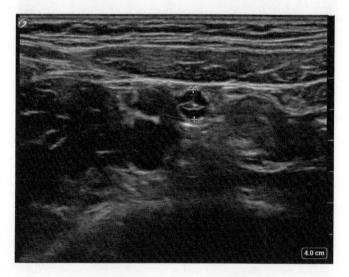

Figure 13.3 Normal appearing appendix visualized in the transverse orientation.

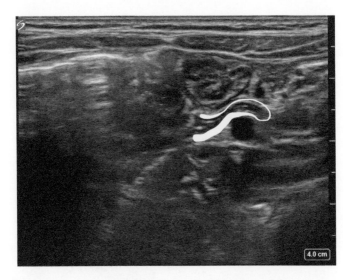

Figure 13.4 Normal appendix in the sagittal orientation. Appendix is a worm-like structure lying directly over the right iliac artery (highlighted).

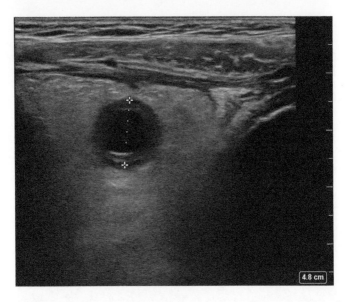

Figure 13.5 Appendicitis. Enlarged appendix with inflammation/stranding surrounding it.

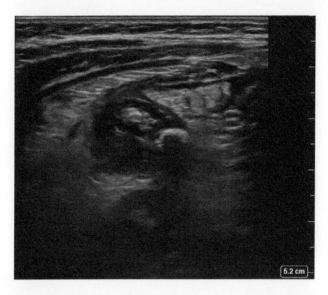

Figure 13.6 Appendicitis. Appendicolith within an enlarged appendix, with surrounding free fluid and tissue inflammation.

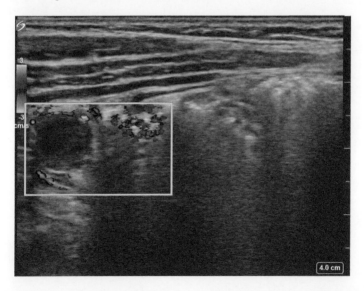

Figure 13.7 Appendicitis. Short-axis view of appendix with color Doppler showing thickened bowel wall vascularity due to inflammation or "ring of fire."

14

Intussusception

INDICATIONS

- Assess patients with episodic abdominal pain, vomiting, and lethargy most commonly at age 4 mo to 4 years old.

PROBE SELECTION

- High-frequency linear transducer.

TECHNIQUE

- Graded compression following the colon from the RLQ→RUQ→LUQ→LLQ using the "lawnmower technique."
- The entire abdomen should be scanned in both longitudinal and transverse planes.
- Look for bowel with very discrete hypoechoic and echogenic layers of edematous mucosa and submucosa.

PEARLS

- Although the ileocolic region is the most common place to find intussusception in children, there is no pattern of distribution in adults.
- Ultrasound features such as the "donut," "target," or "bull's eye" sign, where alternating echogenic bands of mucosa and muscularis and hypoechoic bands of submucosa are visualized in the transverse orientation.
- The transverse orientation may elucidate the edematous layers better.
- In sagittal orientation, you may see a "sandwich," "hayfork sign," or "pseudokidney sign" as you visualize one loop of intestine within the other.

- Small bowel intussusception tends to be smaller (mean diameter 1.5 cm vs. 2.5 for ileocolic).
- Presence of lymph nodes or free fluid within the intussusception is more likely associated with ileocolic.
- Ileocolic intussusception is more commonly found in the right abdomen vs. small bowel intussusception is more commonly found in the periumbilical region and left abdomen.
- False positives can be seen with fecal contents or other conditions that affect bowel wall thickness such as inflammatory bowel disease, infectious enterocolitis, and intramural hematomas.

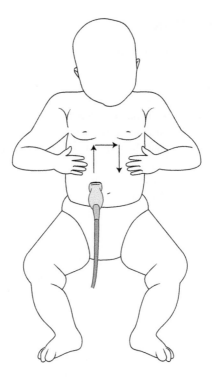

Figure 14.1 Illustration of the graded compression "lawnmower technique."

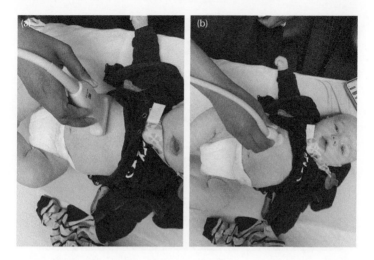

Figure 14.2 Graded compression technique in the transverse (a) and longitudinal (b) orientation.

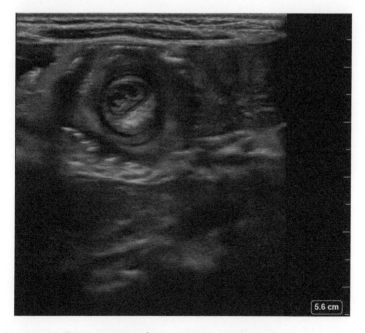

Figure 14.3 Transverse view of intussusception.

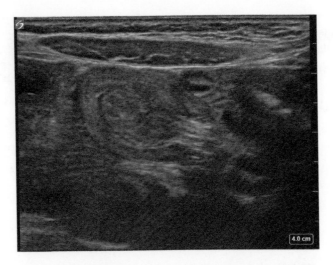

Figure 14.4 Intussusception. "Hayfork sign"; sagittal views of layers of edematous mucosa, muscularis, and submucosa.

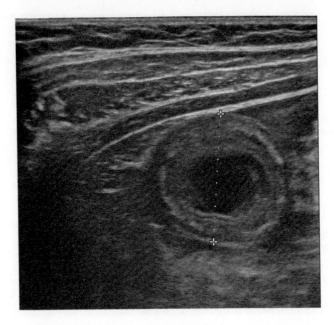

Figure 14.5 Intussusception. Wall-to-wall diameter measurement is approximately 2.1 cm.

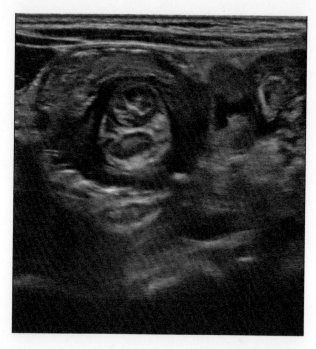

Figure 14.6 Intussusception in transverse orientation with entrapped lymph nodes.

Pylorus

INDICATIONS

- Assess the potential etiology of vomiting in an infant 2–8 weeks of age.

PROBE SELECTION

- High-frequency linear transducer or neonatal low frequency transducer.

TECHNIQUE

- Identify the pylorus by first finding the gallbladder in the short axis.
- Once the gallbladder is identified, the pylorus is usually just medial and posterior to the gallbladder.
- The pylorus can be viewed in either the short or long axis.
- Hypertrophied muscle is hypoechoic while central mucosa will be hyperechoic.
- Pyloric stenosis is defined as a muscle wall thickness >3 mm and pyloric length >15 mm.

PEARLS

- Turn the infant right side down (or left side down if the stomach is markedly distended) if visualization is difficult.
- If the pylorus is difficult to locate, try turning the probe obliquely sagittal to visualize the pylorus longitudinally.

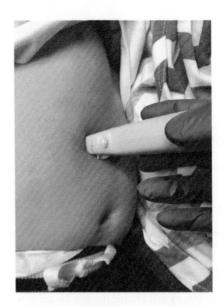

Figure 15.1 Transverse probe placement for identification of pylorus.

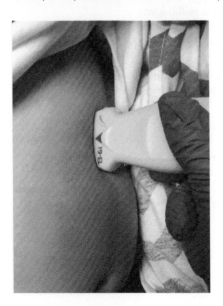

Figure 15.2 Sagittal probe placement for identification of pylorus.

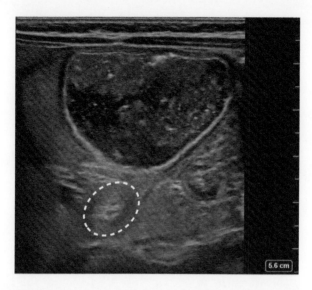

Figure 15.3 Transverse view of the pylorus (circle) with hypertrophic walls. Stomach is anterior.

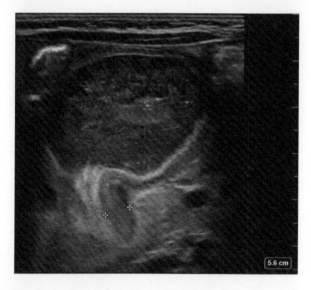

Figure 15.4 Sagittal view of a hypertrophic pylorus (between two plus signs) lying under the stomach.

Biliary

INDICATIONS

- Assess RUQ pain suspicious for cholelithiasis and cholecystitis.

PROBE SELECTION

- 5-1 MHz low-frequency phased array transducer.
- 5-2 MHz low-frequency curvilinear transducer.

TECHNIQUE

- Place the transducer with the indicator toward the patient's head along the mid-clavicular line in the 9th–10th intercostal space.
- Have the patient move into the left lateral decubitus position if the gallbladder is difficult to visualize, or if significant bowel gas is present that obscures view.
- Adjust the probe to create the best long-axis view once the gallbladder has been identified.
- The gallbladder will appear as a pear-shaped, hypoechoic structure with a hyperechoic wall.
- The gallbladder in the long axis can be reliably found by following the main lobar fissure. The main lobar fissure divides the liver into the right and left lobes and connects the gallbladder to the portal vein.
- Look for the "Exclamation Point Sign": In the long axis, the main lobar fissure leading to the gallbladder with the portal vein in short axis creates what looks like an exclamation point.
- Rotate the probe 90° and demonstrate the short axis.
- Measure the gallbladder wall by measuring the diameter from the outer wall to the inner wall.
- Normal gallbladder wall measurement is <3 mm.

- Gallbladder diameter is usually measured in the long axis. Normal gallbladder diameter is <10 cm.
- Pericholecystic fluid may or may not be present in patients with cholecystitis.

Common bile duct
- The normal diameter of the common bile duct is 5 mm or less.
- Common bile duct dilation = >6 mm.

Cholelithiasis
- Gallstones are hyperechoic, mobile structures located within the gallbladder with posterior shadowing.
- Gallstones will appear within the gallbladder with shadowing obscuring the tissues behind.

PEARLS

- Remove excess bowel gas by having the patient lie in the left lateral decubitus position.
- Remember that the common bile duct runs parallel to the portal vein. Place color Doppler on them to distinguish between.
- The duodenum can be mistaken for the gallbladder. Remember that the duodenum is normally next to the liver, has dark outer walls, and is peristaltic. The gallbladder has a bright wall, is surrounded by the liver, and is not peristaltic.
- Side lobe and other types of artifacts and polyps may be mistaken for sludge or gallstones, respectively. Remember that gallstones move when the patient moves, and artifacts will transcend beyond the walls of the gallbladder, where sludge stays squarely within the gallbladder walls.

Pearls 123

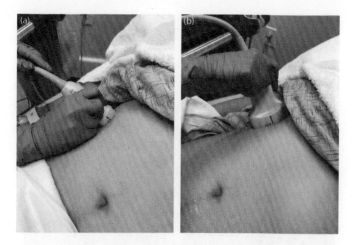

Figure 16.1 Sagittal orientation of the probe in the RUQ. Sweep probe along the costal margin toward the mid-axillary line on the patient's right. A phased array (a) or abdominal probe (b) for larger patients is appropriate.

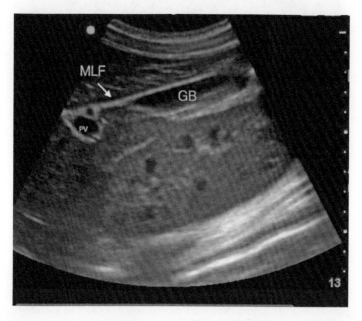

Figure 16.2 Exclamation Point Sign: The gallbladder (GB) is connected to the portal vein (PV) via the main lobar fissure (MLF).

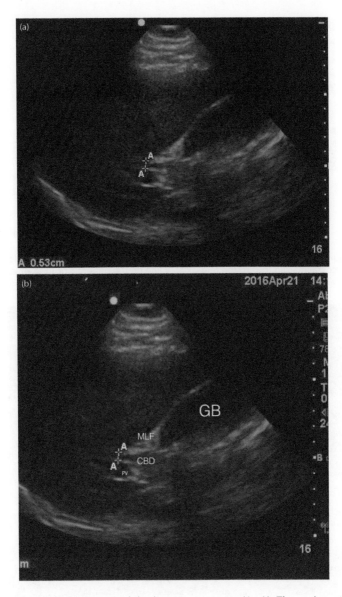

Figure 16.3 (a,b) Common bile duct measurement (A—A). The exclamation point sign is present (GB, PV, and MLF). The common bile duct runs parallel to the portal vein. The diameter of the abnormal common bile duct is >5 mm.

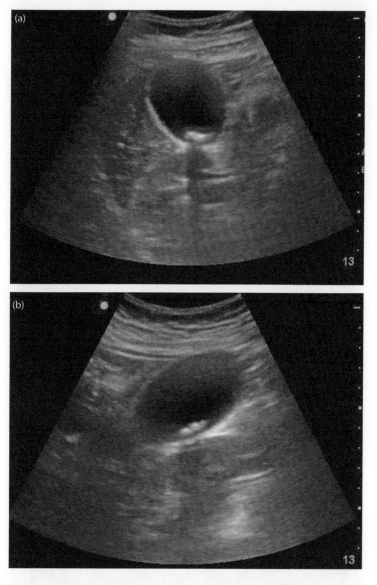

Figure 16.4 (a,b) Gallstones. Hyperechoic gallstones with posterior shadowing. Unlike gallbladder polyps, gallstones move with patient movement.

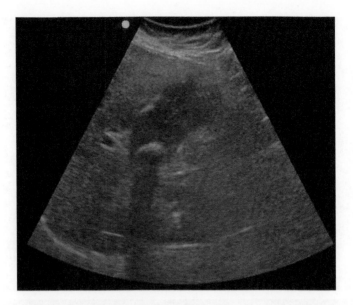

Figure 16.5 Gallstone with posterior shadowing.

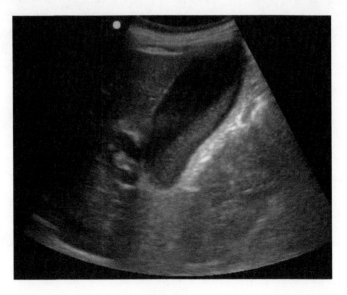

Figure 16.6 Sludge within the gallbladder.

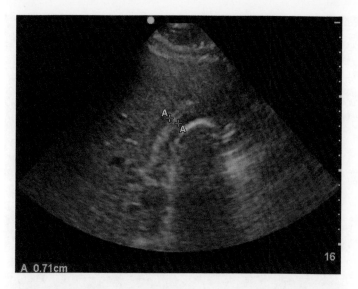

Figure 16.7 WES SIGN. Large gallstone that encompasses entire gallbladder, such that the wall (W), echo of the stone (E), and shadowing are most visible.

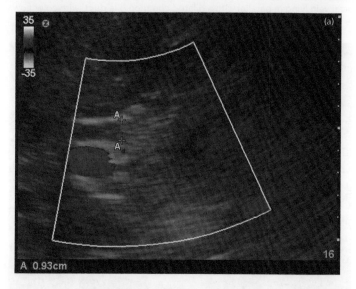

Figure 16.8 (a,b) Common bile duct. Color Doppler showing portal vein lying in parallel with a dilated common bile duct, with color flow in the portal vein and no flow in the bile duct. *(Continued)*

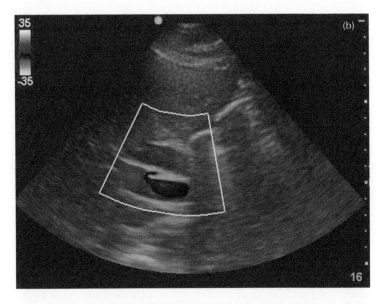

Figure 16.8 (*Continued*) (a,b) Common bile duct. Color Doppler showing portal vein lying in parallel with a dilated common bile duct, with color flow in the portal vein and no flow in the bile duct.

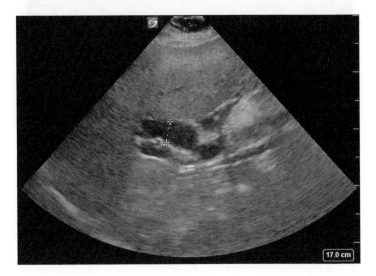

Figure 16.9 Dilated common bile duct.

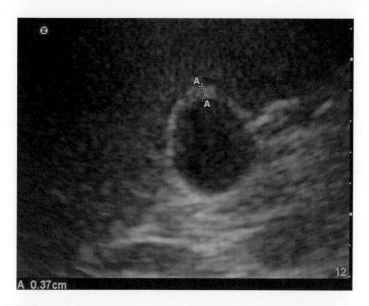

Figure 16.10 Measurement of the gallbladder wall in transverse axis. Gallbladder wall measurement is usually the outer wall to the inner wall.

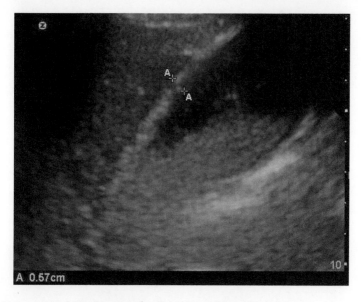

Figure 16.11 Measurement of gallbladder wall in sagittal plane.

PART VI

TRAUMA

17 Focused assessment sonography in trauma (FAST) 133

Focused assessment sonography in trauma (FAST)

INDICATIONS

- Assess active and persistent bleeding in hemodynamically stable patients.
- Evaluate any patient in shock.

PROBE SELECTION

- 5-1 MHz low-frequency phased array transducer.

TECHNIQUE

Right upper quadrant (RUQ)

- Place probe along mid-axillary line in the long axis or along the costal margin on the patient's right. Move the probe up and down the rib spaces until equal parts of the liver and kidney are viewed in the middle of the screen.
- Concentrate on three areas: infra-diaphragmatic space, Morison's pouch (hepatorenal space), and caudal liver tip.
- Fan through the entire space while moving your probe up and down the rib spaces.

Left upper quadrant (LUQ)

- Position probe posterior to the mid-axillary line to avoid obscureness caused by stomach contents.
- Reach over the patient from the right side such that your "knuckles are touching the gurney." This will ensure your probe is placed more posteriorly.
- Move the probe up and down the rib spaces until equal parts of the spleen and kidney are in the middle of the screen.

- Concentrate on two areas: infra-diaphragmatic space, peri-splenic space.
- Angle the probe diagonally such that the probe face is nestled within the intercostal space to eliminate rib shadows.

Suprapubic view

- Place probe between the umbilicus and pubic symphysis in both the transverse and sagittal planes.
- Angle the probe in the transverse orientation such that the probe face is aimed toward the patient's feet and toward the pubic symphysis.
- Fan the probe right to left in the sagittal orientation
- Fan the probe cephalad to caudad in the transverse orientation.
- Fluid will collect superiorly and posterior to the bladder; in women, fluid can collect behind the uterus and in the virtual space between the bladder and uterus anteriorly.

Cardiac view: Subxiphoid

- Place the probe just below xiphoid process, marker to the patient's right
- Use the liver as an acoustic window to obtain a four-chamber view of the heart

PEARLS

- Small, subtle, fluid pockets may accumulate in the sub-diaphragmatic space, liver or splenic tips before larger, more obvious free fluid accumulates. Ensure full visualization of these areas in the RUQ and LUQ views.
- Ensure your "knuckles are on the bed" in the LUQ view. Place the probe more superiorly and posteriorly such that the sonographer's knuckles are touching the patient bed.
- Angle the probe face such that it is nestled parallel to the ribs within the intercostal space to avoid rib shadows.
- Allow the liver to act as an acoustic window to better visualize the heart. Aim the probe first toward the liver and slowly fan toward the patient's left shoulder at a 45° angle to allow the heart to appear.
- The bladder can be reliably found if the probe is placed directly superior to the suprapubic bone, with the probe face pointing posteriorly and down toward the patient's feet.

Pearls 135

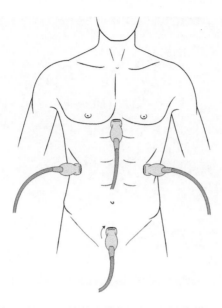

Figure 17.1 Four main areas of the FAST.

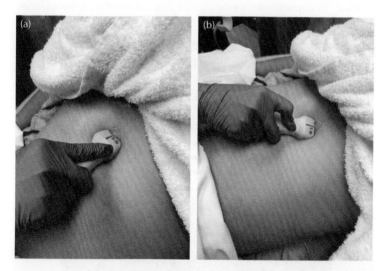

Figure 17.2 Subxiphoid probe placement. Aim probe face toward the patient's right shoulder or head (a) and slowly fan probe toward the patient's left shoulder at a 45° angle to visualize the heart (b).

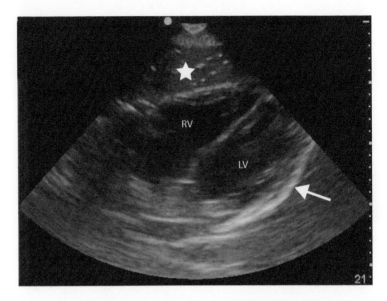

Figure 17.3 Subxiphoid view of the heart. A small part of the liver can be seen at the top left of the screen (star). Ventricles are located at the top of the screen (labeled). The hyperechoic border surrounding the heart is the pericardium (arrow).

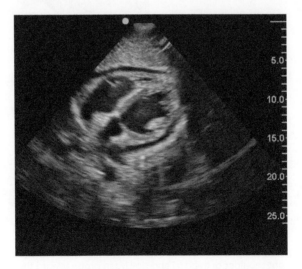

Figure 17.4 Pericardial effusion. Circumferential fluid surrounding the heart.

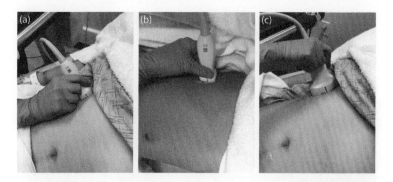

Figure 17.5 The RUQ views can be obtained either by the anterior approach (a), moving toward the patient's right costal margin and mid-axillary line; or (b) starting directly at the mid-axillary line. For larger patients, the abdominal probe can be used for the FAST exam (c).

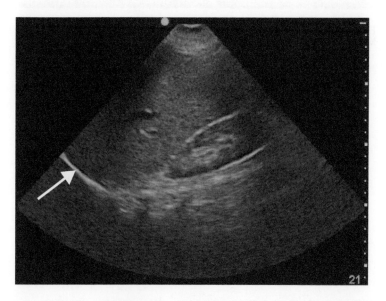

Figure 17.6 Normal RUQ view. Liver (left) and kidney (right). Note how in the normal lung, the thoracic spine (hyperechoic, scalloped line) meets the diaphragm (a thin, smooth hyperechoic line), and does not move past it (white arrow). In the presence of a normal air-filled lung, the visualization of the spine stops once it meets the diaphragm.

138 Focused assessment sonography in trauma (FAST)

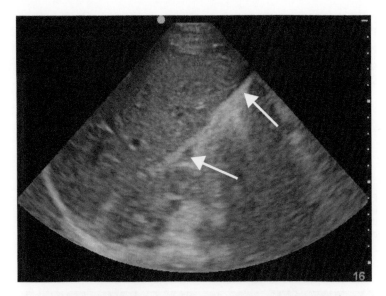

Figure 17.7 Subtle pocket of anechoic, free fluid at the tip of the liver and in Morrison's pouch (white arrows).

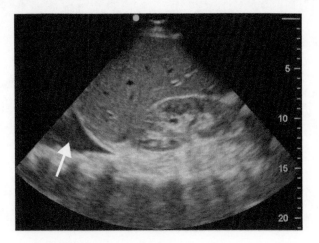

Figure 17.8 RUQ view. Fluid accumulation located *above* the diaphragm indicating the presence of free fluid in the thorax (white arrow). In the presence of a normal air-filled lung, the visualization of the spine stops once it meets the diaphragm. The presence of a pleural effusion or hemothorax allows for the spine to be visualized in its entirety across the screen, past the diaphragm. This is called the *spine sign*.

Pearls 139

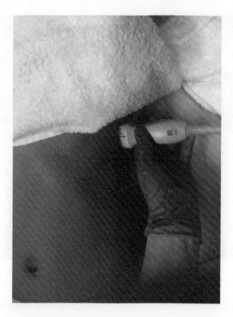

Figure 17.9 Placement of probe in the LUQ. Knuckles are touching the gurney so that the probe is positioned posteriorly.

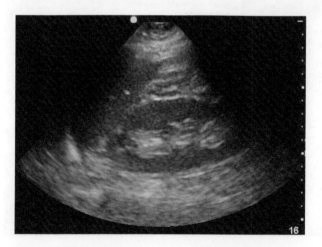

Figure 17.10 Normal LUQ view. Spleen is located on the left screen. Kidney appears in the middle of the screen. Splenorenal space in between the kidney and spleen.

140 Focused assessment sonography in trauma (FAST)

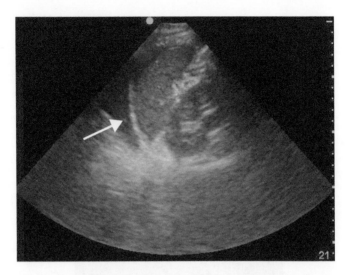

Figure 17.11 Small free fluid pocket along the tip of the spleen. Notice another anechoic fluid collection above the diaphragm in the thorax (white arrow) on the left side of the screen. This fluid collection is in the pleura, not the abdomen.

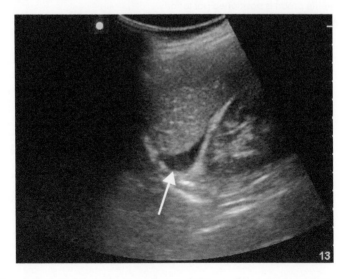

Figure 17.12 Fluid pocket along the sub-diaphragmatic space moving toward the spleno-renal space (white arrow).

Pearls 141

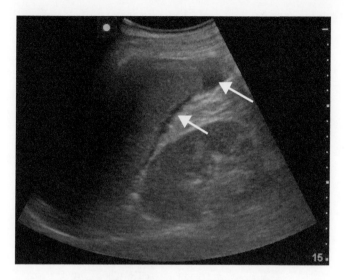

Figure 17.13 Fluid along the tip of the spleen and in the splenorenal space (white arrows).

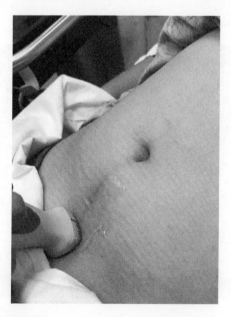

Figure 17.14 Suprapubic view in transverse orientation.

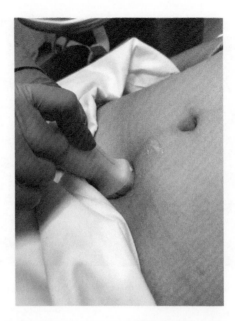

Figure 17.15 Suprapubic view in sagittal orientation.

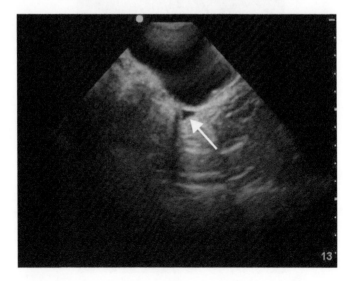

Figure 17.16 Sagittal view of the bladder with a small triangular fluid pocket posterior to the bladder (white arrow).

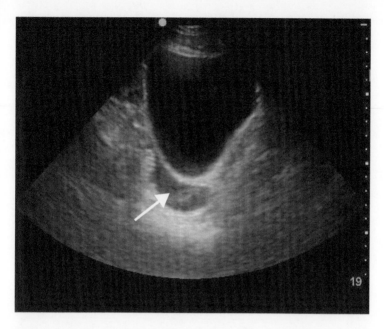

Figure 17.17 Transverse view of the bladder with a sizeable fluid pocket posterior to the bladder (white arrow).

PART VII

RENAL, URINARY, AND REPRODUCTIVE SYSTEMS

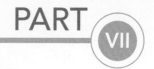

18 Renal	147
19 First trimester pregnancy	157
20 Testicular	165

PART

Renal

INDICATIONS

- Assess for presence of hydronephrosis in patients suspected of having renal colic.
- Evaluate bladder volume prior to catheterization.

PROBE SELECTION

- 5-1 MHz low-frequency phased array transducer.
- 5-2 MHz low-frequency curvilinear transducer.

TECHNIQUE

- Evaluate RUQ (refer to FAST RUQ) to view the right kidney.
- Place probe over the right anterior axillary line at the level of the xiphoid process in the long axis.
- Using liver as the acoustic window, scan the right kidney in the long axis looking for hydronephrosis (anechoic fluid originating in renal sinus).
- Rotate probe 90° clockwise to scan the kidney in the short axis.
- Evaluate LUQ (refer to FAST LUQ) to view the left kidney.
- Place probe over the left posterior axillary line at the level of the xiphoid process in the long axis.
- Fan inferiorly to avoid scanning through bowel gas.
- Scan the left kidney in the long axis looking for hydronephrosis.
- Rotate probe 90° clockwise to scan the kidney in the short axis.
- Evaluate pelvis via the suprapubic view (transverse view in FAST pelvis) to evaluate bladder volume.
- Place probe over the suprapubic area in the transverse orientation, fanning down into the pelvis.

PEARLS

- Renal views are obtained in a similar fashion to the RUQ and LUQ views in the FAST. However, the focus is on the kidney and not the liver and spleen.
- The right kidney may be better viewed by starting with the probe in the mid-axillary line, to bypass gas and abdominal contents.
- Renal vasculature can be mistaken for mild hydronephrosis. Place color Doppler on the kidney to check for flow.
- Renal cysts can be mistaken for severe hydronephrosis. Cysts develop from the parenchyma, whereas hydronephrosis develops from the collecting system within the central part of the kidney.
- Bladder volume can be measured by measuring the length × width × height × 0.52.

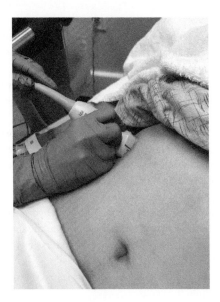

Figure 18.1 Sagittal orientation of the probe in RUQ, starting more anteriorly on the abdomen and moving the probe laterally along the costal margin.

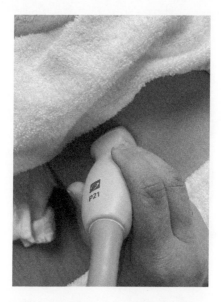

Figure 18.2 Transverse orientation of the probe in RUQ.

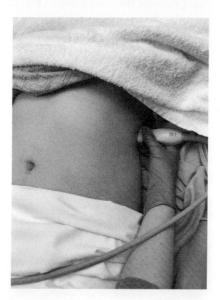

Figure 18.3 Sagittal orientation of the probe in the LUQ.

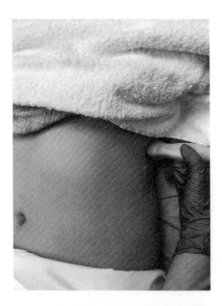

Figure 18.4 Probe in the transverse orientation. Placement of probe is similar to that of the FAST LUQ; however, the focus is only on the kidney.

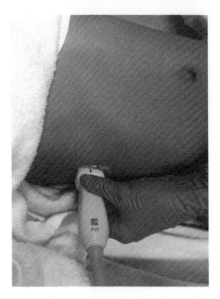

Figure 18.5 Sagittal orientation of the probe for visualization of the right kidney. Start along the costal margin or along the mid-axillary line.

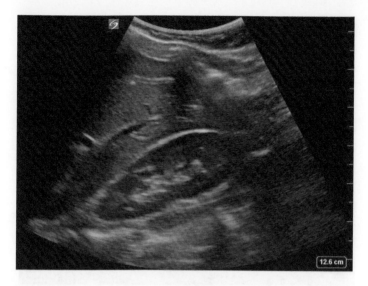

Figure 18.6 Normal sagittal view of the kidney in the RUQ.

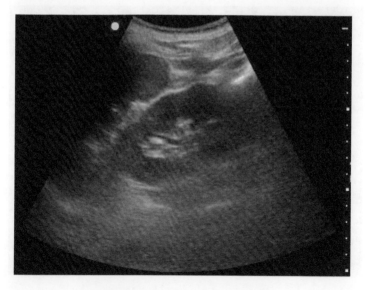

Figure 18.7 Normal sagittal view of the kidney in the LUQ.

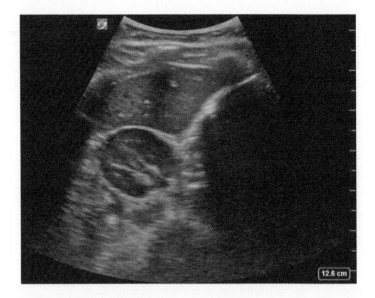

Figure 18.8 Normal transverse view of the kidney.

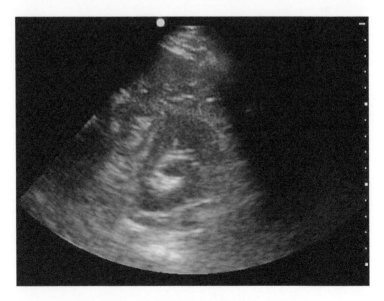

Figure 18.9 Transverse view of the kidney. Mild hydronephrosis.

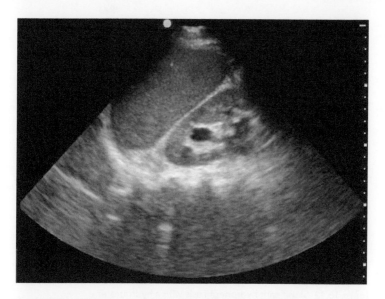

Figure 18.10 Sagittal view of the kidney. Mild hydronephrosis.

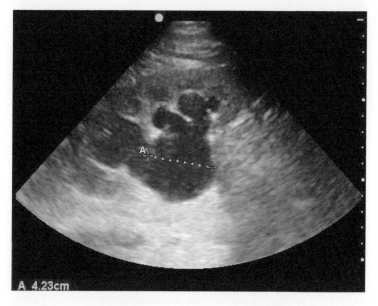

Figure 18.11 Moderate hydronephrosis with a significant hydroureter.

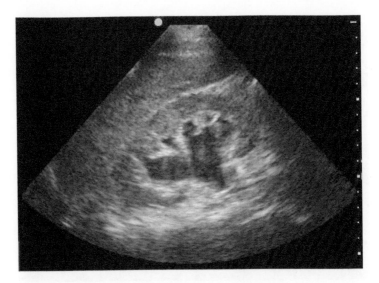

Figure 18.12 Significant hydronephrosis with a hydroureter.

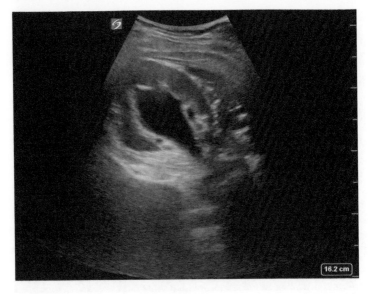

Figure 18.13 Hydronephrosis with the destruction of the renal sinus, with a hydroureter.

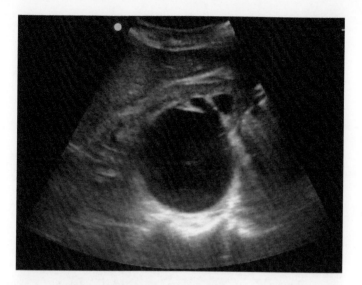

Figure 18.14 Severe hydronephrosis with destruction of the renal parenchyma. Hydronephrosis can be distinguished from a renal cyst in that it originates from the central part of the kidney.

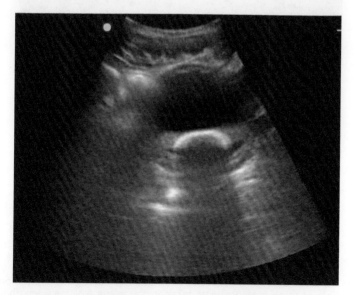

Figure 18.15 Transverse view of the bladder with bladder stone present.

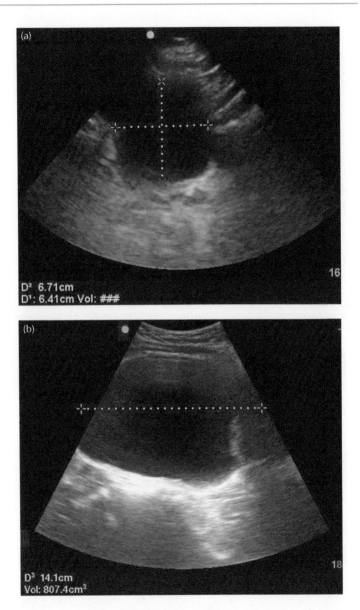

Figure 18.16 Bladder in transverse orientation (a) and sagittal orientation (b). Two of three measurements taken in this plane (volume = length × width × height × 0.52).

First trimester pregnancy

INDICATIONS

- Determine the presence of intrauterine pregnancy (IUP).
- Determine dating by crown rump length (CRL).
- Evaluate fetal heart rate (FHR).
- Determine the presence of free peritoneal fluid.

PROBE SELECTION

- 5-2 MHz low-frequency curvilinear probe (for transabdominal).
- 8-5 MHz high-frequency intra-cavity probe (for transvaginal).

TECHNIQUE

Transabdominal

- Place the transducer in the suprapubic region in the sagittal plane (as seen in the FAST exam). The uterus is posterior to the bladder. Move, rock, and fan the probe, interrogating the entire uterus first, then assess the endometrium for evidence of an IUP. Rotate the probe to 90° so that transducer is in the transverse axis, then fan the cephalad to caudad.
- Look for evidence of an IUP, which is a sac-like structure with a yolk sac and/or fetal pole.
- If a fetal pole is present, measure CRL by finding the longest dimension and placing the calipers on the crown and rump. If >7 weeks, fetal cardiac activity should be present (look for flickering in the middle of the thorax).
- Measure FHR if present: in OB mode place M-mode cursor over cardiac activity and under calculations measure peak-to-peak or trough-to-trough for rate.

Transvaginal

- Have the patient empty the bladder, cover transducer per institutional policy. Water-based lubricant is recommended for use on patients.
- Place transducer at the introitus in sagittal orientation with the probe marker pointing anteriorly. Slowly insert into vagina until uterus is visualized on the screen, then gently fan left to right, interrogating the entire uterus. Rotate the probe 90° so the transducer is in coronal (transverse axis) orientation. The probe marker should be pointing toward the patient's right. Fan anterior to posterior.
- Look for evidence of IUP and free fluid. If IUP is present, measure CRL and FHR.

PEARLS

- Perform the transabdominal view first (with a full bladder) and then have the patient empty the bladder if a transvaginal ultrasound is necessary.
- Transabdominal views of the uterus are best visualized with a full bladder because it acts as an acoustic window for the uterus and other surrounding structures.
- Perform a transvaginal ultrasound if an intrauterine pregnancy is not visualized on transabdominal views.
- Positioning is key. When performing a transvaginal ultrasound, the patient should be on a gynecological exam bed, with hips and buttocks at the very edge of the bed. This will allow appropriate positioning of the probe when used in the coronal orientation.
- Make sure you visualize the entire uterus in both planes when looking at the endometrium for evidence of an intrauterine pregnancy to ensure full visualization of the endometrial sac and its contents.
- Remember that the uterus is not always midline. Having to move the probe to the patient's left or right to visualize the uterus is not uncommon.
- Any patient who is in her first trimester based on her last menstrual period who presents with abdominal pain and vaginal bleeding should receive an ultrasound to look for the presence/absence of an intrauterine pregnancy.
- Patients who present with abdominal pain, vaginal bleeding, a positive pregnancy test, and an absence of an intrauterine pregnancy with free peritoneal/pelvic fluid on ultrasound are considered at high risk for ectopic pregnancy until proven otherwise.

Pearls 159

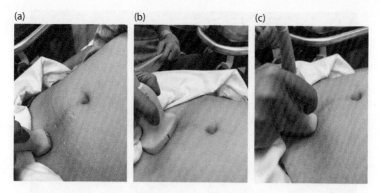

Figure 19.1 Transverse placement (a) and sagittal placement (b) of probe in the suprapubic region. Sagittal placement of probe (c). Notice how the probe is not always placed in the midline. The location of the uterus will not uncommonly be located off midline.

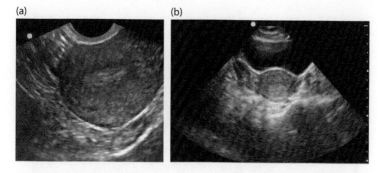

Figure 19.2 Transverse views of the uterus. (a) In this transvaginal view the uterus shows the hyperechoic endometrial stripe in the center of the uterus. (b) In this transabdominal view the uterus with bladder lying anteriorly.

160 First trimester pregnancy

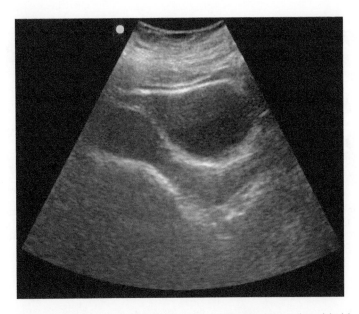

Figure 19.3 Sagittal view of the uterus, including the hypoechoic bladder anterior to the uterus.

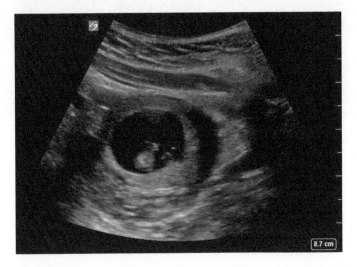

Figure 19.4 Intrauterine pregnancy viewed in the transverse orientation. The yolk sac, a faint, circular ring located to the anatomical left of the IUP, is present.

Pearls 161

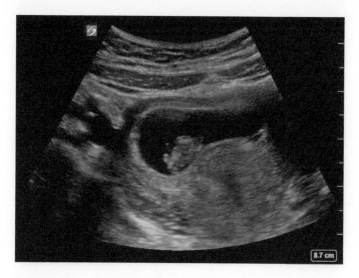

Figure 19.5 Intrauterine pregnancy.

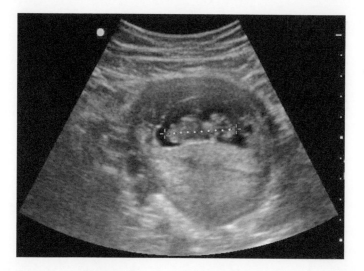

Figure 19.6 Transverse view of uterus with intrauterine pregnancy and crown rump length measurements.

162 First trimester pregnancy

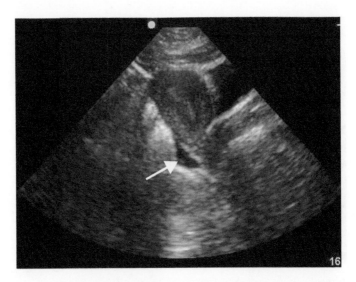

Figure 19.7 Sagittal view of the uterus without the presence of an intrauterine pregnancy, and free fluid (white arrow) in the retrovesicular space. In patients with a positive pregnancy test, vaginal bleeding, and abdominal pain, ectopic pregnancy must be considered.

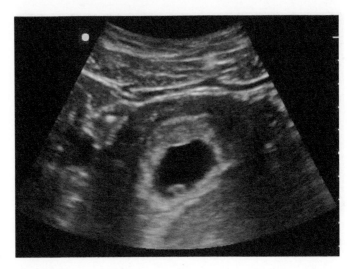

Figure 19.8 Yolk sac. A hyperechoic ring with an anechoic center is an early sonographic sign of pregnancy.

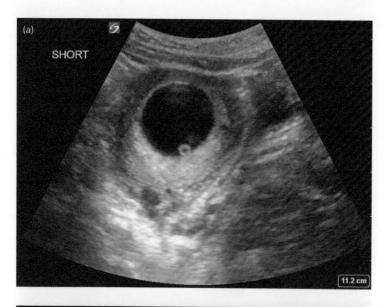

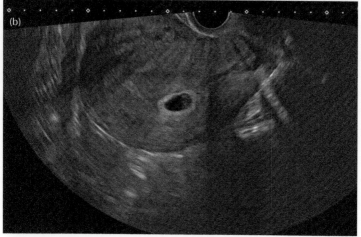

Figure 19.9 (a,b) Intrauterine pregnancy with hyperechoic ring (yolk sac) inside the gestational sac.

Testicular

INDICATIONS

- Assess acute scrotal pain and evaluate for signs of testicular torsion.

PROBE SELECTION

- High-frequency linear transducer.

TECHNIQUE

- Have patient sit with ankles crossed and use towel to support scrotum and penis.
- Place the transducer with the indicator toward the patient's right on the unaffected hemiscrotum.
- Obtain transverse views of each testicle.
- Place the transducer with the indicator toward the patient's right.
- Rotate the probe to 90° and obtain sagittal views of each testicle.
- Place the transducer with the indicator toward the patient's head.
- Obtain a side by side midline view of both testes for comparison of power flow.
- Difference in flow between each testicle is concerning for torsion.
- Use spectral Doppler to assess for both venous and arterial flow in both testes.
- Resistive index = RI > 0.75 is concerning for early or incomplete torsion.

PEARLS

- While scanning the unaffected side, it is important to calibrate the power Doppler settings on the healthy hemiscrotum (increase gain until noise is present; then decrease color gain until it just disappears).

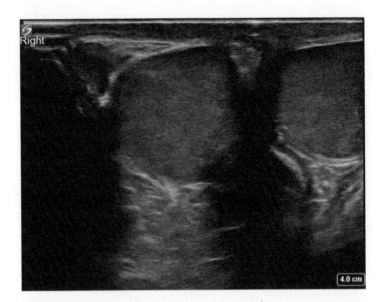

Figure 20.1 Normal testicles.

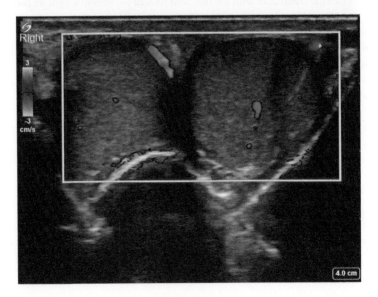

Figure 20.2 Normal testicles with normal flow.

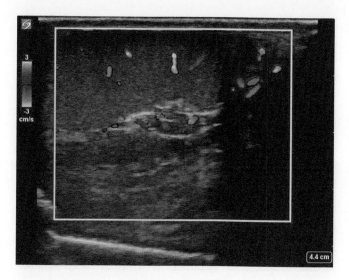

Figure 20.3 Normal testicle with normal flow.

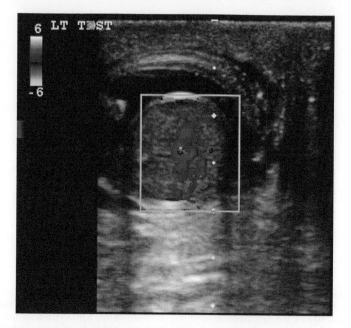

Figure 20.4 Testicle with increased flow.

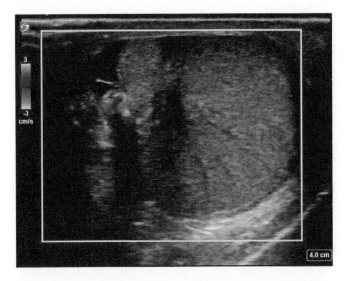

Figure 20.5 Testicle with no flow.

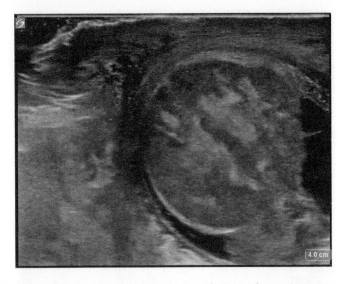

Figure 20.6 Testicular torsion. Key ultrasound findings of testicular torsion are the absence of normal blood flow, elevated resistive index (RI > 0.75), increase in the size of the testis and epididymis, homogeneous echotexture in early torsion, and heterogeneous echotexture in late torsion, and reactive hydrocele in some cases.

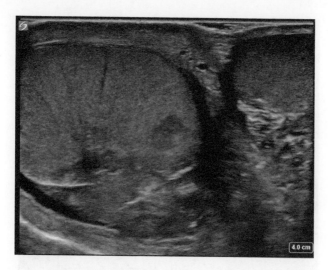

Figure 20.7 Testicular torsion. Hypoechoic regions can represent necrosis. Hyperechoic regions can represent hemorrhage if reperfusion is present.

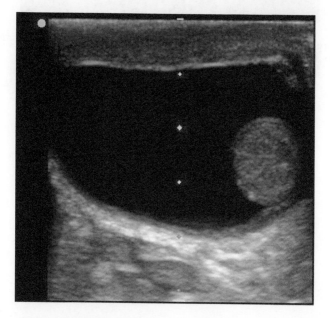

Figure 20.8 Hydrocele in a neonate.

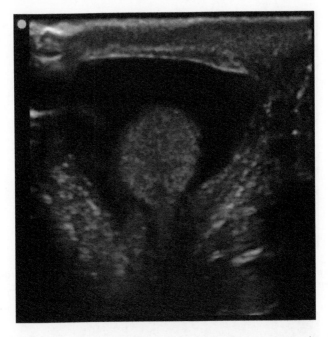

Figure 20.9 Hydrocele, noted as a simple fluid collection surrounding the testis.

PART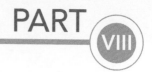

PROCEDURAL

21	Femoral nerve block	173
22	Intraosseous placement	179
23	Lumbar puncture	183
24	Endotracheal tube confirmation	189
25	Peripheral intravenous placement	193
26	Upper extremity nerve blocks	199
27	Central line placement	207

Femoral nerve block

INDICATIONS

- To control pain from femoral neck and mid-shaft fractures.
- To provide anesthesia for procedures on anterior and medial thigh.

CONTRAINDICATIONS

- Refrain on patients with altered mental status, neurologic deficits, infection at the injection site.

PROBE SELECTION

- High-frequency linear transducer.

PRE-PROCEDURE CHECKLIST

- Remember that this procedure blocks both motor and sensory (takes out quad).
- Document a good neurological exam prior to the procedure.
- Perform an informed consent and address fall risk.
- Confirm the consultant is amenable to the procedure.
- Place on monitors and be wary of anesthetic systemic toxicity.

TECHNIQUE

- Perform procedure in full sterile technique by draping the patient, using a sterile probe cover, sterile lube, and sterile gloves.
- Place probe in transverse orientation 1 cm distal to inguinal ligament.
- Identify femoral artery (anechoic pulsating vessel), located just lateral to artery.

- Note that femoral nerve will be a hyperechoic, honeycombed structure lateral to artery, located under hyperechoic fascia iliaca.
- Use in-plane technique to visualize the needle continuously, instilling local anesthetic above and below the nerve.
- Dose 0.5 mL/kg of 0.25% bupivacaine (adult dose is 15–20 mL).
- Inject the area around the nerve. Do not inject the nerve itself.

PEARLS

- Remember that the femoral nerve and the femoral artery are in two separate compartments that are separated by two fascial planes called the fascia lata and fascia iliaca. The needle should pass through the fascia iliaca in order to appropriately deliver the block.
- Stay clear of all vascular structures or lymph nodes.
- Needle should never touch the nerve (anesthetic injected around nerve).
- There should be no resistance when injecting the anesthetic. If there is resistance, pull back and start again.

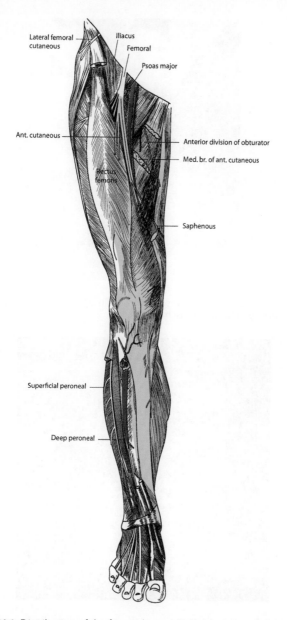

Figure 21.1 Distribution of the femoral nerve (light blue). (Image courtesy of Dr. Jason Fischer.)

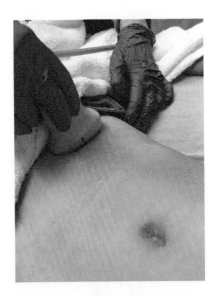

Figure 21.2 Placement of ultrasound in groin to view the femoral nerve. (Image courtesy of Dr. Jason Fischer.)

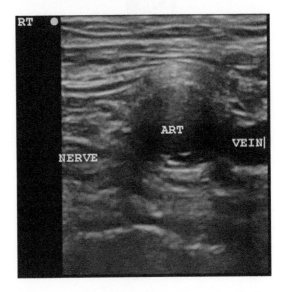

Figure 21.3 Transverse orientation of the probe to view the femoral nerve, which is located adjacent to the femoral artery. (Image courtesy of Dr. Jason Fischer.)

Pearls 177

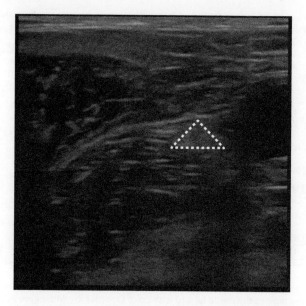

Figure 21.4 Transverse view of the femoral nerve (triangle). Femoral nerve is nestled in a different fascial plane than the femoral vein and artery. In order to appropriately block the femoral nerve, the needle must move through the fascia iliaca. (Image courtesy of Dr. Jason Fischer.)

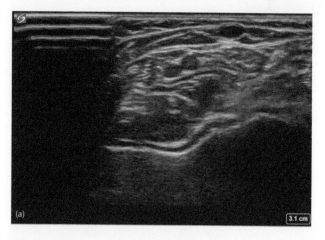

Figure 21.5 Femoral vein is adjacent to the femoral artery. View the artery next to the nerve (a) and with color Doppler (b), with nerve adjacent to the artery. The nerve has a honeycomb appearance. (Image courtesy of Dr. Jason Fischer.) *(Continued)*

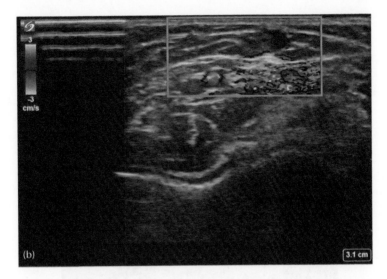

Figure 21.5 (*Continued*) Femoral vein is adjacent to the femoral artery. View the artery next to the nerve (a) and with color Doppler (b), with nerve adjacent to the artery. The nerve has a honeycomb appearance. (Image courtesy of Dr. Jason Fischer.)

Intraosseous placement

INDICATIONS

- Confirm intraosseous (IO) placement during patient resuscitation.

PROBE SELECTION

- High-frequency linear transducer.

TECHNIQUE

- Place the probe immediately proximal or distal to the IO site and visualize the bone in the sagittal plane.
- Use color Doppler and watch for turbulence as saline is administered in the interosseous space.
- If no flow is visualized, switch to power Doppler.
- Rotate the probe in transverse orientation and repeat.
  - If flow is present in interosseous space, the needle is in the correct space.
  - If flow is outside the interosseous space, replace the line.

PEARLS

- In infants you can go through and through and still see some flow in the interosseous space on ultrasound.
- If ding a check after fluids have been infusing, need to use power doppler to detect flow.

180 Intraosseous placement

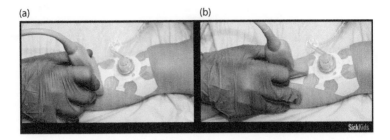

Figure 22.1 Placement of probe in the transverse orientation (a) and sagittal orientation (b) to confirm correct intraosseous infusion. (Image courtesy of Dr. Jason Fischer.)

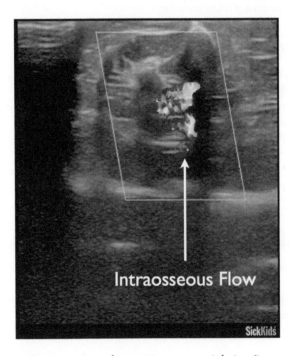

Figure 22.2 Transverse view of correct intraosseous infusion. (Image courtesy of Dr. Jason Fischer.)

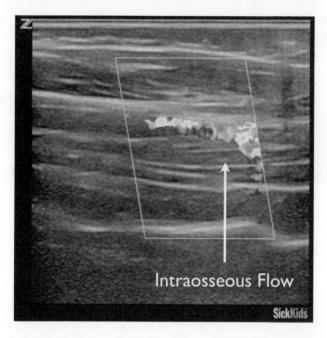

Figure 22.3 Sagittal view of correct intraosseous infusion. (Image courtesy of Dr. Jason Fischer.)

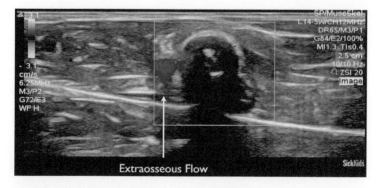

Figure 22.4 Transverse view of extraosseous flow indicating incorrect intraosseous infusion placement. (Image courtesy of Dr. Jason Fischer.)

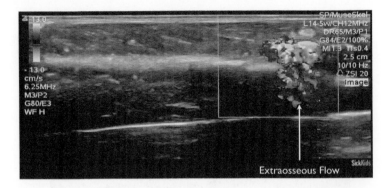

Figure 22.5 Sagittal view of extraosseous flow indicating incorrect intraosseous infusion placement. (Image courtesy of Dr. Jason Fischer.)

Lumbar puncture

INDICATIONS

- Identification of spinal landmarks prior to performance of lumbar puncture.

PROBE SELECTION

- High-frequency linear transducer.

TECHNIQUE

- Position probe indicator pointing toward patient's head.
- Locate the sacrum.
- Move cranially to locate the L4/L5 interspace and place probe in the middle of the patient's back (so that it presents to the middle of the screen).
- Ultrasound will show spinous processes in cross section with the intervertebral space in between.
- Mark this interspace making a horizontal line from the center of the probe.
- Rotate probe indicator pointing toward the patient's right.
- Locate the spinous process and align it in the center of your screen.
- Ultrasound screen will show the spinous process in the middle of the back if the probe is directly on top of the spinous process. This represents the true midline of the spine.
- Mark the true midline making a vertical line from the center of your probe.
- The intersection of these lines indicates the insertion site for LP.

PEARLS

- Use a curvilinear transducer in large patients.
- You can measure the depth to the intervertebral space in order to estimate the length of needle you will need.

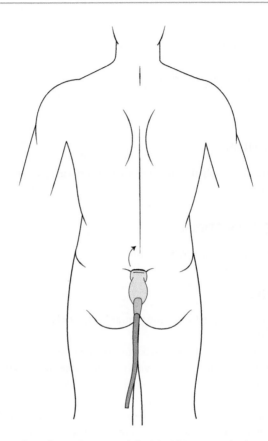

Figure 23.1 Place the probe around the L4−L5 intervertebral space in both the transverse and sagittal orientation.

Pearls 185

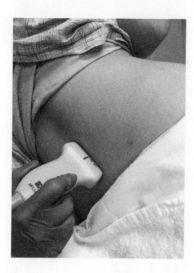

Figure 23.2 Sagittal orientation. Probe marker is pointing toward the patient's head, which exposes the spinous processes and the intervertebral space in between.

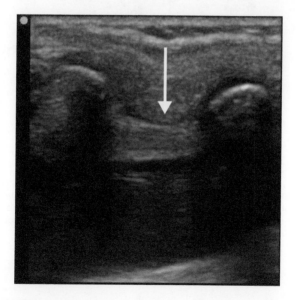

Figure 23.3 Sagittal view of the spinous processes and the intervertebral space (white arrow) in between.

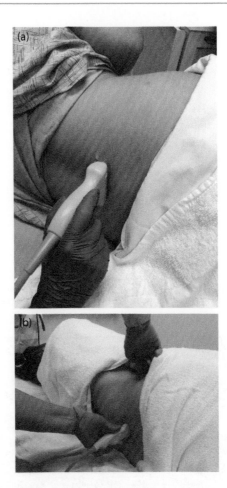

Figure 23.4 (a) Transverse orientation. Probe marker points toward the patient's right or left. Probe should be placed directly over the spinous process. The center of the spinous process should align with the center of the probe face. This will denote the middle of the screen. (b) Palpate the superior border of the posterior iliac crest to ensure proper placement of probe over correct lumbar spinous processes.

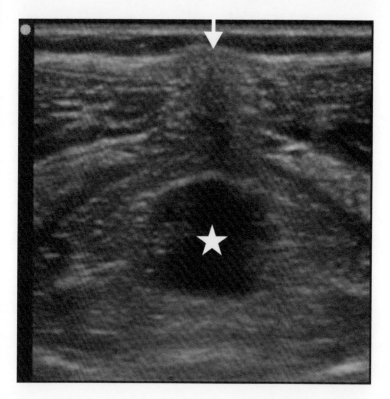

Figure 23.5 Transverse view of the spinous process of an infant in the top middle screen (white arrow). The spinous process denotes the patient's midline. The spinal canal (star) is seen in the far field as an anechoic circle.

Endotracheal tube confirmation

INDICATIONS

- Confirm proper endotracheal tube placement.

PROBE SELECTION

- High-frequency linear transducer.

TECHNIQUE

- With the patient's neck in slight extension, place the linear transducer in the transverse orientation (indicator toward the patient's right), in the middle of the neck, and scan cephalad starting at the suprasternal notch.
- The trachea will appear as a hypoechoic structure with a bright echogenic line, which represents air in the trachea.
- The esophagus appears as a collapsed oval structure posterior and to the anatomical left of the trachea.

PEARLS

- If the endotracheal tube is in the esophagus, you will see a "double trachea" sign in which the propped open esophagus appears similar to the trachea.
- If the endotracheal tube is in the trachea, you will see no change in the ultrasound view.

190 Endotracheal tube confirmation

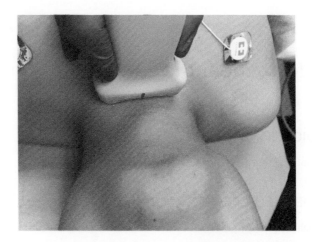

Figure 24.1 Transverse placement of the ultrasound probe on the neck.

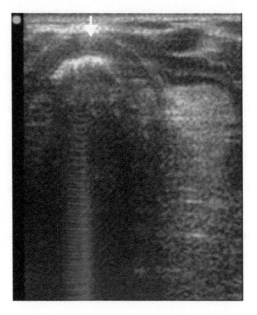

Figure 24.2 Tracheal ultrasound after endotracheal intubation. Endotracheal tube is located in the trachea. The esophagus, located adjacent to the trachea on the right of the screen, is empty.

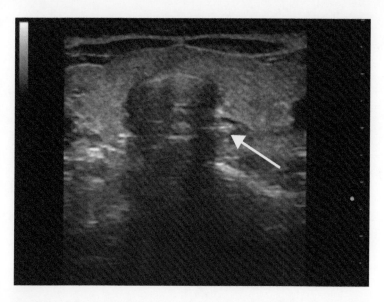

Figure 24.3 Esophageal intubation. Esophagus is now visible on screen right (arrow), with empty trachea.

25

Peripheral intravenous placement

INDICATIONS

- Expose peripheral veins in patients with difficult peripheral vascular access.

PROBE SELECTION

- High-frequency linear transducer.

TECHNIQUE

- Lay patient supine, arm abducted and ventral surface of upper arm exposed, tourniquet applied near axilla.
- Set up the US machine so it is directly across the gurney in direct line of sight.
- Scan area between the forearm to proximal humerus for a good target vein.
- Target big, superficial veins with a straight course.
- Basilic, brachial, and cephalic are popular veins in the arm.
- Once target vessel is located, hold US probe in non-dominant hand and the angiocatheter in the dominant hand.
- Place vessel (in short axis is preferred) in the middle of the screen so the vessel is directly under the middle of the transducer.
- Use the center of the probe as a reference and insert the needle at a 30°–45° angle so that the tip of the needle intersects the vein directly under the transducer.
- It may be necessary to advance the transducer as the needle is advanced in order to keep the needle and vein in the center of the screen.
- The needle should appear as an echogenic dot, or there may be secondary signs of the needle including ring down artifact or tenting of venous wall.
- Once there is blood return in the catheter, place the transducer to the side and proceed with catheter advancement.

PEARLS

- Although it may be easier to attempt a peripheral IV via the transverse orientation, the advantage of peripheral IV attempts via the sagittal orientation is that the needle can be visualized going through the entire length of the vein; a disadvantage is that the neighboring structures cannot be seen in this orientation.
- Remember that veins and arteries are easily compressible in the arm. Try to avoid any pressure. Use color Doppler when evaluating vessels.
- Use a 1.88 in angiocatheter for deep peripheral veins. The standard angiocatheters are not long enough.

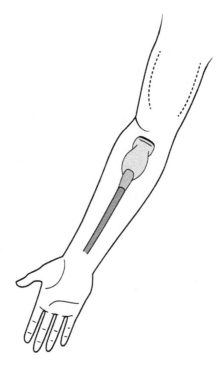

Figure 25.1 Place probe in the transverse orientation directly over the antecubital fossa or puncture site with tourniquet applied.

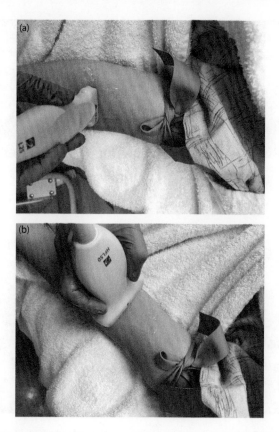

Figure 25.2 (a,b) Visualize veins with tourniquet applied. The transverse orientation of the probe provides the most probe stability on the arm.

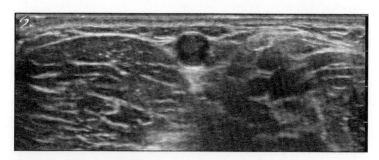

Figure 25.3 Transverse view of the peripheral vein, approximately 0.5 cm deep.

196 Peripheral intravenous placement

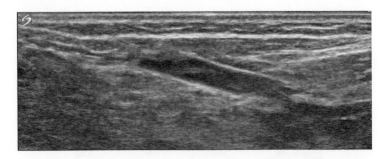

Figure 25.4 Sagittal view of the peripheral vein.

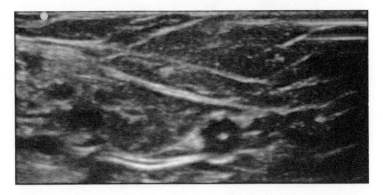

Figure 25.5 Confirmation of needle (hyperechoic dot within the hypoechoic circle) within the vein. Transverse view.

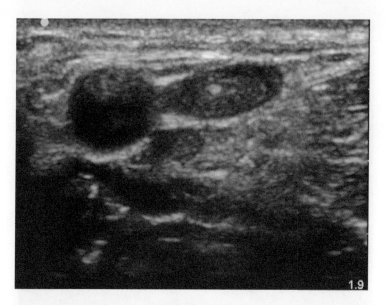

Figure 25.6 Peripheral line confirmation. Artery and adjacent vein (ovoid and slightly compressed) with angiocatheter within the vein.

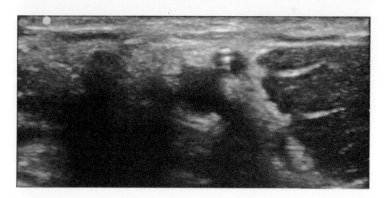

Figure 25.7 Transverse view of needle in the peripheral vein with ring down artifact.

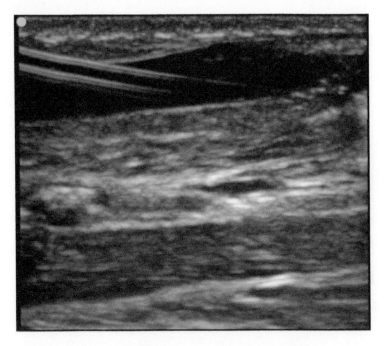

Figure 25.8 Sagittal view of the peripheral vein with IV in place.

Upper extremity nerve blocks

INDICATIONS

- To control pain and provide anesthesia for hand procedures.

PROBE SELECTION

- High-frequency linear transducer (small or larger footprint).

TECHNIQUE

Radial nerve block

- Place probe transversely at the crease of the wrist on radial side and identify the radial artery (pulsating anechoic vessel).
- Ensure that the radial nerve, a small, hyper-echoic structure with a honeycomb appearance, is on the radial or lateral side of the artery.
- Trace radial nerve up to mid-forearm, where it will course away from the artery.
- Prep skin, use a clear adhesive or sterile probe cover, and sterile lube.
- Use the in-plane technique to advance needle (25 g should suffice) toward the nerve and inject 3–5 cc local anesthetic around the nerve, aiming for circumferential spread around the nerve.

Ulnar nerve block

- Place the probe transversely at the crease of the wrist on the ulnar side and identify the ulnar artery (pulsating anechoic vessel).
- Ensure that the ulnar nerve, a small, hyper-echoic, honeycombed structure, is on the ulnar or medial side of the artery.
- Trace the ulnar nerve up to the mid-forearm, where it will course away from the artery.
- Prepare the skin, using a clear adhesive, or sterile probe cover, and sterile lube.

- Use the in-plane technique to advance needle toward nerve and inject 3–5 cc of local anesthetic around the nerve, aiming for circumferential spread.
- Flex the elbow and externally rotate wrist for optimal positioning of ultrasound probe.

Median nerve block

- Place probe in the transverse orientation on the mid-forearm volar surface; the median nerve will be a hyper-echoic, honeycombed structure sandwiched between the muscle bellies of flexor digitorum profundus and flexor digitorum superficialis.
- Prepare the skin, using a clear adhesive or sterile probe cover, and sterile lube.
- Use the in-plane technique to advance the needle toward the nerve and inject 3–5 cc local anesthetic around the nerve, aiming for circumferential spread.
- Median nerve is most easily located in the mid-forearm, where it stands alone.

PEARLS

- The radial nerve branches at the level of the wrist, so a block at the level of the forearm, below, or at the radial styloid process is recommended.
- The radial nerve runs along the "radial" or lateral side of the artery.
- The medial nerve is best viewed at the mid-forearm, where it is larger, standing alone.
- The median nerve can easily be mistaken for a tendon at the level of the wrist, so move the probe proximally to confirm the location of the nerve.
- The ulnar nerve is located along the ulnar side (medial) to the artery.
- Nerves can have the artifact of anisotropy, where the nerve appears darker or lighter depending on the angle of the probe on the skin.

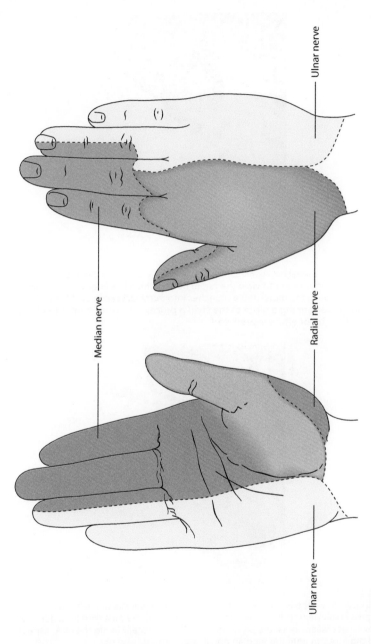

Figure 26.1 Nerve distribution of hand.

202 Upper extremity nerve blocks

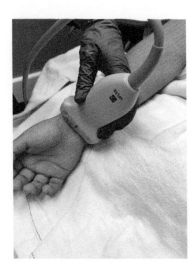

Figure 26.2 Radial nerve. Place the probe slightly lateral to the midline in the transverse orientation to view the radial nerve, which lies lateral to the radial artery. Because the radial nerve branches into terminal branches at the level of the wrist, performing a block at the styloid process at the wrist or at the level of the forearm or elbow is preferred.

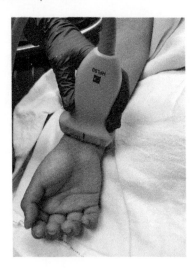

Figure 26.3 Median nerve. Place the probe in the middle of the forearm in the transverse orientation. Because tendons can easily be mistaken for a nerve at the wrist crease, move the probe proximally and distally along the volar aspect of the forearm until the median nerve is confirmed.

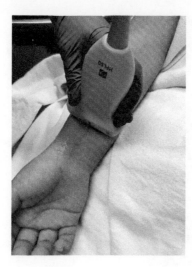

Figure 26.4 Median nerve. Move proximally with the probe in the middle of the forearm to improve visualization of the median nerve.

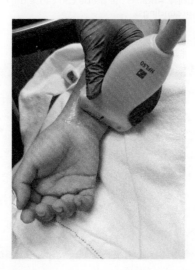

Figure 26.5 Ulnar nerve. The probe is placed in the transverse orientation medial to the midline. The ulnar nerve runs medial to the ulnar artery from the mid-forearm to the wrist.

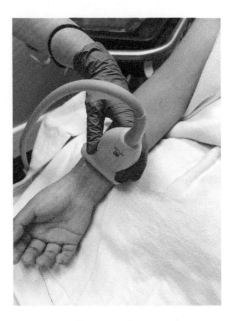

Figure 26.6 Anisotropy. Angling the probe can cause the nerve to be darker or lighter than its surroundings.

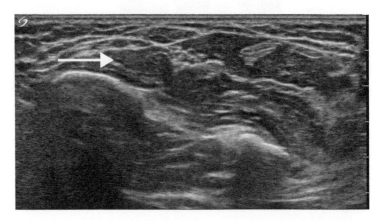

Figure 26.7 Median nerve in mid-forearm in the transverse orientation (middle of the screen in nearfield). The median nerve has a honey-combed, hyperechoic appearance and is best visualized in the mid-forearm (arrow).

Pearls 205

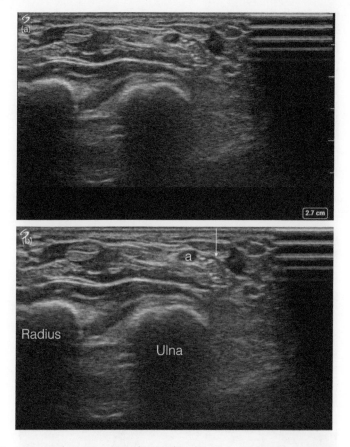

Figure 26.8 Ulnar artery (a) and nerve (b) (white arrow). Transverse orientation.

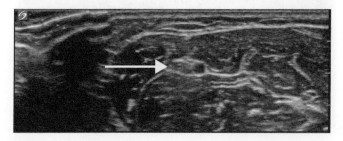

Figure 26.9 Ulnar artery and adjacent ulnar nerve (white arrow).

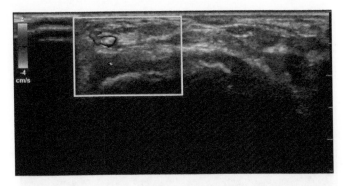

Figure 26.10 Radial artery. To confirm location, place color Doppler on the artery.

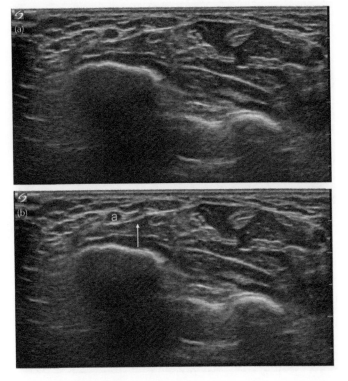

Figure 26.11 (a,b) Radial artery (a) and nerve (white arrow). The radial nerve at the wrist is located adjacent to the radial artery, superficial to the radius.

Central line placement

INDICATIONS

- Improves visualization of vessel and surrounding structures.
- Decreases risk of arterial and nerve puncture and improves first pass success of venous cannulation.

PROBE SELECTION

- High-frequency linear probe.
- Sterile central venous catheter tray.
- Sterile probe cover and sterile gel, betadine.

TECHNIQUE

- Central line placement can be performed via the static technique or dynamic technique. In the static technique, the vein is seen on ultrasound but the procedure is performed without the ultrasound. Dynamic technique requires the utilization of ultrasound throughout the entire procedure.
- If using dynamic technique for central line placement, the ultrasound probe should be in the non-dominant hand, leaving the dominant hand to perform the procedure.
- Note the location of the artery, vein, nerve, and any other pertinent structures, such as wires, masses, anatomical variation.
    - Femoral vein
        - Know the anatomical landmarks in the groin from medial to lateral: lymph, vein, artery, nerve.
        - Palpate the groin for the artery and place the ultrasound probe on the skin directly on top.

- Move the probe cephalad so that the artery and vein are adjacent. As vessels move distally, the artery tends to move posterior to the vein.
  - Internal jugular
    - Know the anatomical landmarks in the neck, including the heads of the sternocleidomastoid muscle, just above the clavicle. The apex of these heads forms a triangle, which can be palpated when the patient moves his head to the opposite side.
    - The internal jugular is located beneath the heads of the sternocleidomastoid muscle. Palpate the carotid artery and triangle apex and put the ultrasound probe on the skin directly on top of the apex.
- Place probe in the transverse orientation with the vein centered in the middle of the screen.
- Move the needle a few millimeters distal to the probe, and at a 45° angle, puncture the skin until the needle tip is seen on the screen.
- As the needle tip is advanced, move the probe away from the needle by a few millimeters in order to keep the tip of the needle in view.

PEARLS

- For internal jugular venous cannulation, place the patient in Trendelenburg to increase the size of the vein.
- Betadine can be used as a conductive medium if sterile ultrasound gel is not available.
- If using the static technique, use the ultrasound again to ensure the threaded wire is in the correct vessel prior to dilating.
- Prior to starting the procedure, place the ultrasound machine such that the insertion site is between the sonographer and the screen.
- Set up the sterile probe cover, gel, and the patient in sterile fashion prior to dressing in a sterile gown. This includes putting non-sterile gel on the linear probe so that it is ready when the sterile probe cover is placed over it.
- Remember that the middle of the probe corresponds to the middle of the screen. If the needle is inserted into the skin from the middle of the screen, you will see the needle enter from the middle of the screen.
- Use the push and advance technique with the needle to keep the tip of the needle visualized during the procedure.

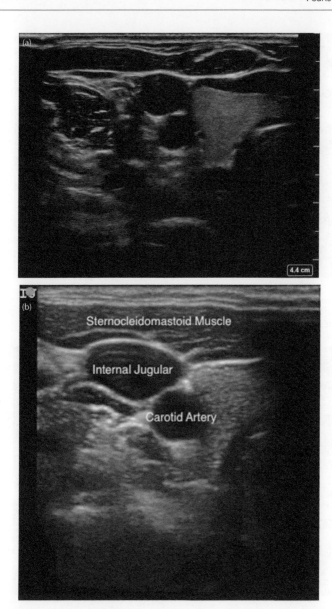

Figure 27.1 Transverse view of internal jugular vein (a and b), located anterior to artery, confirmed by color Doppler (c). The internal jugular vein is located approximately 1 cm deep to the skin. *(Continued)*

210 Central line placement

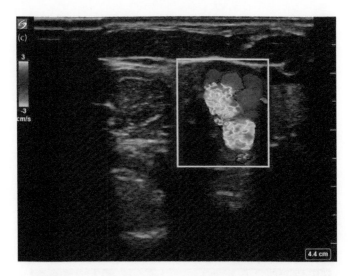

Figure 27.1 (*Continued*) Transverse view of internal jugular vein (a and b), located anterior to artery, confirmed by color Doppler (c). The internal jugular vein is located approximately 1 cm deep to the skin.

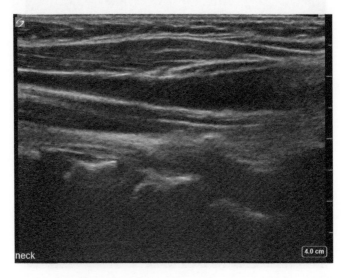

Figure 27.2 Sagittal view of the internal jugular (compressed at one end) and a partial view of the carotid posterior to the internal jugular vein. The needle would enter from the left screen (if the probe indicator was pointing toward the patient's head).

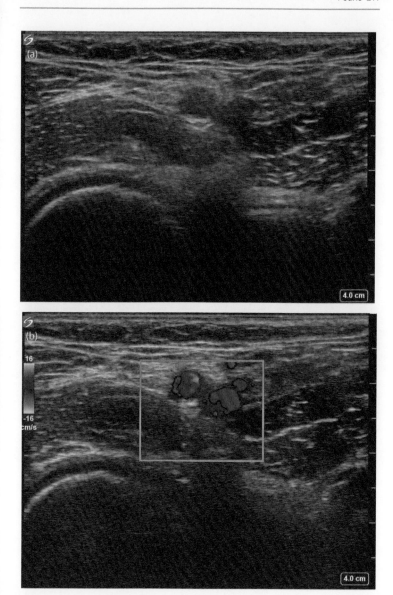

Figure 27.3 Transverse views of the femoral artery and vein. Vessels without color Doppler (a). Vessels with color Doppler (b).

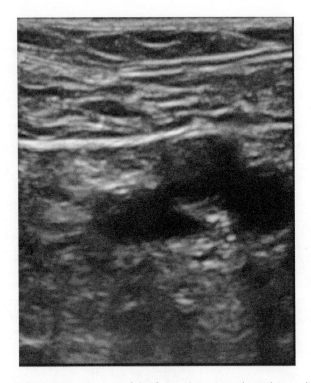

Figure 27.4 Transverse views of the femoral artery and vein lying adjacent to one another. Using color Doppler and compression can help differentiate between the two vessels.

PART IX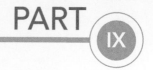

NERVOUS SYSTEM

28 Ocular   215

Ocular

INDICATIONS

- Evaluate patients with history or exam concerning for elevated intracranial pressure, foreign body, retinal detachment, or vitreous pathology.

PROBE SELECTION

- High-frequency linear transducer.

TECHNIQUE

- Gently place a sterile, clear adhesive dressing over the patient's closed eye.
- Place a copious amount of ultrasound gel on the adhesive dressing.
- Place the probe indicator *temporally* in the transverse orientation and toward the forehead in the sagittal orientation.
- Anchor your scanning thumb on the bridge of the patient's nose.
- Scan in two planes:
  - Transverse plane = probe indicator pointing temporally on the patient fanning cephalad to caudad; have patient move eyes left to right during exam.
  - Sagittal plane = probe indicator pointing toward forehead, fanning left to right; have patient move eyes cephalad to caudad during the exam.

NOTES

- Optic nerve sheath diameter measurement can be performed when elevated intracranial pressure is suspected. Measure 0.3 cm posterior from where the optic nerve enters the globe and at that level measure diameter across the optic nerve. Abnormal diameter is >0.5 cm.

- Retinal detachment has the appearance of a thick, hyperechoic cord that is tethered to the optic nerve posteriorly and will move within the vitreous during a kinetic exam.
- Posterior vitreous detachments are thin, loosely adherent strands that will move freely within the vitreous during a kinetic exam.
- "Mac-on" retinal detachments are a true emergency and require stat ophthalmologic evaluations. The macula is located around 5 mm lateral (temporal) to the optic nerve. Mac-on retinal detachments are retinal detachments where the macula is still attached and the central visual acuity is still preserved. Ultrasound shows the retina on the temporal side is still attached at the optic nerve and detaches *distal to* the macula.
- "Mac-off" retinal detachments refer to a retinal detachment where the macula has detached and central visual acuity is not preserved. Ultrasound shows the retina on the temporal side detaches at the optic nerve *before it reaches the macula* so that it is only tethered to the back of the eye by the optic nerve.
- Kinetic exam: when the probe is still on the patient's eyelids but the patient's eyes are moving.

PEARLS

- Increase the gain when evaluating the vitreous to improve visualization of changes within the vitreous.
- Decrease the gain when evaluating the optic nerve, which allows differentiation between the nerve and surrounding soft tissue.
- Ensure you do not put pressure on the eye with your scanning hand by anchoring your fingers/thumb on the bridge of the nose and cheekbone.
- The optic nerve diameter can be inaccurate if measured at the wrong angle. Make every effort to try to measure the nerve when captured in the correct plane.
- Remember that the macula is located on the temporal side of the eye. Ensure that the probe is always positioned with the probe indicator pointing temporally so that you can reliably know if the macula is still attached with suspected retinal detachments.

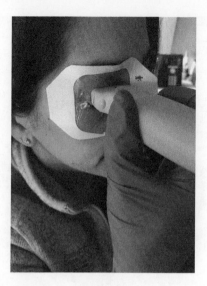

Figure 28.1 Transverse orientation with the probe indicator pointing temporally. Rest pinky finger to the patient's nose to decrease pressure on the patient's face.

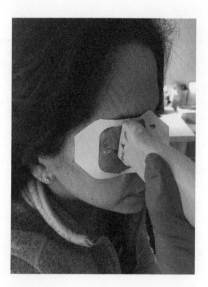

Figure 28.2 Sagittal orientation with probe indicator pointing upward.

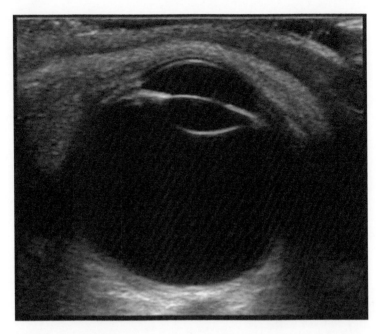

Figure 28.3 Normal eye.

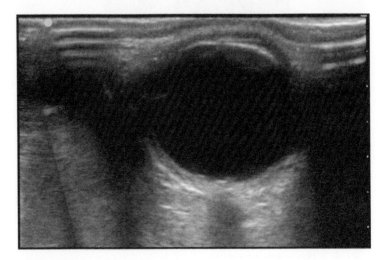

Figure 28.4 Normal vitreous.

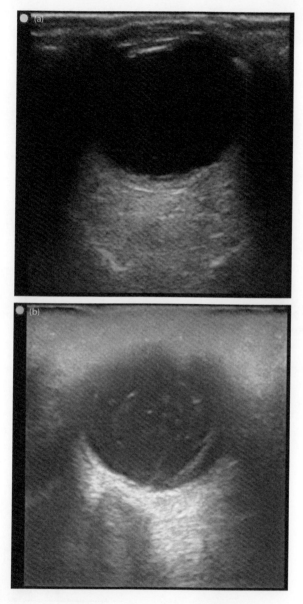

Figure 28.5 Ocular ultrasound of the same eye. Vitreous is incompletely viewed due to poor gain (a). The same eye viewed with increased gain (b) shows the presence of vitreous contents (hemorrhage).

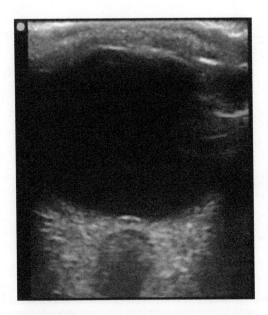

Figure 28.6 Optic nerve sheath appears as a hypoechoic column posterior to the eye.

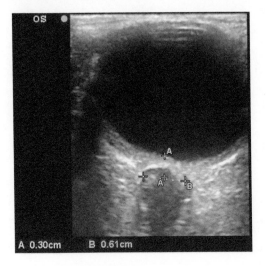

Figure 28.7 Measurement of optic nerve sheath. Measure 3 mm distal to the juncture of the retina to the optic nerve (A) and measure the diameter of the sheath (B). Diameters >5 mm are considered abnormal.

Pearls 221

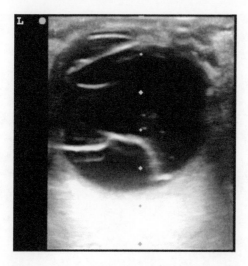

Figure 28.8 Retinal detachment. Detached retina is a hyperechoic and ribbon-like structure that is tethered to the optic nerve, and moves with dynamic movements of the eye.

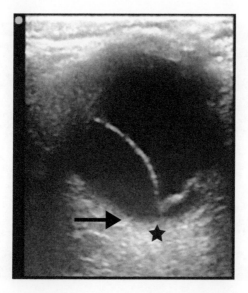

Figure 28.9 Mac-off retinal detachment. Optic nerve (blue star). Macula (black arrow). Retina is completely detached, tethered only to the optic nerve.

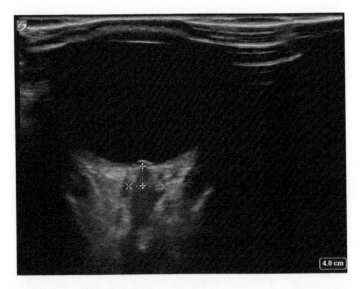

Figure 28.10 Papilledema. Note the elevation of the optic disk from the retina.

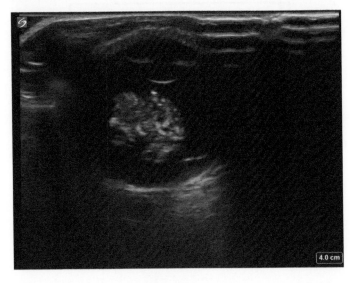

Figure 28.11 Retinoblastoma. Note echogenic calcifications wthin the mass coming from the retina.

Bibliography

Adhikari S, Blaivas M. Utility of bedside sonography to distinguish soft tissue abnormalities from joint effusions in the emergency department. *J Ultrasound Med*. 2010;29:519–26.

American College of Emergency Physicians. Definition of Clinical Ultrasonography [policy statement]. Approved January 2014. Accessed May 7, 2018 at https://www.acep.org/patientcare/policy-statements/definition-of-clinical-ultrasonography.

Anderson KL, Jenq KY, Fields JM et al. Diagnosing heart failure among acutely dyspneic patients with cardiac, inferior vena cava, and lung ultrasonography. *Am J Emerg Med*. 2013;31:1208–14.

Barbier C, Loubières Y, Schmit C et al. Respiratory changes in inferior vena cava diameter are helpful in predicting fluid responsiveness in ventilated septic patients. *Intensive Care Med*. 2004;30:1740–6.

Barsuk JH, Cohen ER, Vozenilek JA. Simulation-based education with mastery learning improves paracentesis skills. *J Grad Med Educ*. 2012;4:23–7.

Barsuk JH, McGaghie WC, Cohen ER. Simulation-based mastery learning reduces complications during central venous catheter insertion in a medical intensive care unit. *Crit Care Med*. 2009;37:2697–701.

Bartocci M, Fabrizi G, Valente I et al. Intussusception in childhood: Role of sonography on diagnosis and treatment. *J Ultrasound*. 2015;18:205–11.

Blaivas M. Bedside emergency department ultrasonography in the evaluation of ocular pathology. *Acad Emerg Med*. 2000;7:947–50.

Blaivas M, Fox J. Outcome in cardiac arrest patients found to have cardiac standstill on the bedside emergency department echocardiogram. *Acad Emerg Med*. 2001;8:616–21.

Blaivas M, Lyon M, Duggal S. A prospective comparison of supine chest radiography and bedside ultrasound for the diagnosis of traumatic pneumothorax. *Acad Emerg Med*. 2005;12:844–9.

Damewood S, Jeanmonod D, Cadigan B. Comparison of a multimedia simulator to a human model for teaching FAST exam image interpretation and image acquisition. *Acad Emerg Med*. 2011;18:413–9.

Das SK, Choupoo NS, Haldar R et al. Transtracheal ultrasound for verification of endotracheal tube placement: A systematic review and meta-analysis. *Can J Anaesth.* 2015;62:413–23.

Deanehan J, Gallagher R, Vieira R et al. Bedside hip ultrasonography in the pediatric emergency department: A tool to guide management in patients presenting with limp. *Pediatr Emerg Care.* 2014;30:285–7.

Fields JM, Fischer JI, Anderson KL et al. The ability of renal ultrasound and ureteral jet evaluation to predict 30-day outcomes in patients with suspected nephrolithiasis. *Am J Emerg Med.* 2015;33:1402–6.

Freeman K, Dewitz A, Baker WE. Ultrasound-guided hip arthrocentesis in the ED. *Am J Emerg Med.* 2007;25:80–6.

Gallagher RA, Levy J, Vieira RL et al. Ultrasound assistance for central venous catheter placement in a pediatric emergency department improves placement success rates. *Acad Emerg Med.* 2014;21:981–6.

Gallard E, Redonnet JP, Bourcier JE et al. Diagnostic performance of cardiopulmonary ultrasound performed by the emergency physician in the management of acute dyspnea. *Am J Emerg Med.* 2015;33:352–8.

Garcia-Pena BM, Taylor GA, Fishman SJ et al. Costs and effectiveness of ultrasonography and limited computed tomography for diagnosing appendicitis in children. *Pediatrics.* 2000;106:672–6.

Gaspari RJ, Horst K. Emergency ultrasound and urinalysis in the evaluation of flank pain. *Acad Emerg Med.* 2005;12:1180–4.

Geria RN, Raio CC, Tayal V. Point-of-care ultrasound: Not a stethoscope-a separate clinical entity. *J Ultrasound Med.* 2015;34:172–3.

Goodman A, Perera P, Mailhot T et al. The role of bedside ultrasound in the diagnosis of pericardial effusion and cardiac tamponade. *J Emerg Trauma Shock.* 2012;5:72–5.

Gottlieb M, Bailitz J. Can transtracheal ultrasonography be used to verify endotracheal tube placement? *Ann Emerg Med.* 2015;66:394–5.

Gottlieb M, Bailitz JM, Christian E et al. Accuracy of a novel ultrasound technique for confirmation of endotracheal intubation by expert and novice emergency physicians. *West J Emerg Med.* 2014;15:834–9.

Jang TB, Ruggeri W, Dyne P et al. Learning curve of emergency physicians using emergency bedside sonography for symptomatic first-trimester pregnancy. *J Ultrasound Med.* 2010;29:1423–8.

Kanji HD, McCallum J, Sirounis D et al. Limited echocardiography-guided therapy in subacute shock is associated with change in management and improved outcomes. *J Crit Care.* 2014;29:700–5.

Karacabey S, Sanrı E, Gencer EG et al. Tracheal ultrasonography and ultrasonographic lung sliding for confirming endotracheal tube placement: Faster? Reliable? *Am J Emerg Med.* 2016;34.

Kendall JL, Shimp RJ. Performance and interpretation of limited right upper quadrant ultrasound by emergency physicians. *J Emerg Med.* 2001;21(1):7–13.

Kilker BA, Holst JM, Hoffmann B. Bedside ocular ultrasound in the emergency department. *Eur J Emerg Med.* 2014;21:246–53.

Kuhn M, Bonnin RL, Davey MJ et al. Emergency department ultrasound scanning for abdominal aortic aneurysm: Accessible, accurate, and advantageous. *Ann Emerg Med.* 2000;36:219–23.

Labovitz AJ, Noble VE, Bierig M et al. Focused cardiac ultrasound in the emergent setting: A consensus statement of the American Society of Echocardiography and American College of Emergency Physicians. *J Am Soc Echocardiogr.* 2010;23:1225–30.

Lam SH, Grippo A, Kerwin C et al. Bedside ultrasonography as an adjunct to routine evaluation of acute appendicitis in the emergency department. *West J Emerg Med.* 2014;15:808–15.

Li Y, Wang J, Wei X. Confirmation of endotracheal tube depth using ultrasound in adults. *Can J Anaesth.* 2015;62:832.

Lichtenstein DA, Mezière GA, Lagoueyte JF et al. A-lines and B-lines: Lung ultrasound as a bedside tool for predicting pulmonary artery occlusion pressure in the critically ill. *Chest.* 2009;136:1014–20.

Ma OJ, Mateer JR, Ogata M et al. Prospective analysis of a rapid trauma ultrasound examination performed by emergency physicians. *J Trauma.* 1995;38:879–85.

Machare-Delgado E, Decaro M, Marik PE. Inferior vena cava variation compared to pulse contour analysis as predictors of fluid responsiveness: A prospective cohort study. *J Intensive Care Med.* 2011;26:116–24.

Mallin M, Craven P, Ockerse P et al. Diagnosis of appendicitis by bedside ultrasound in the ED. *Am J Emerg Med.* 2015;33:430–2.

Mandavia DP, Aragona J, Childs J et al. Prospective evaluation of standardized ultrasound training for emergency physicians. *Acad Emerg Med.* 1999;6:382.

Mandavia DP, Hoffner R, Mahaney K et al. Bedside echocardiography by emergency physicians. *Ann Emerg Med.* 2001;38:377–82.

Marin JR, Lewiss RE, AAP et al. Point-of-care ultrasonography by pediatric emergency medicine physicians. *Pediatrics.* 2015;135(4):e1113–22.

Marshburn TH, Legome E, Sargsyan A et al. Goal-directed ultrasound in the detection of longbone fractures. *J Trauma.* 2004;57:329–32.

Melniker LA, Leibner E, McKenney MG et al. Randomized controlled clinical trial of point-of care, limited ultrasonography for trauma in the emergency department: The first sonography outcomes assessment program trial. *Ann Emerg Med.* 2006;48:227–35.

Mendiratta-Lala M, Williams T, de Quadros N et al. The use of a simulation center to improve resident proficiency in performing ultrasound-guided procedures. *Acad Radiol.* 2010;17:535–40.

Miller AH, Pepe PE, Brockman CR et al. ED ultrasound in hepatobiliary disease. *J Emerg Med.* 2006;30:69–74.

Min YG, Lee CC, Bae Y et al. Accuracy of sonography performed by emergency medicine residents for the diagnosis of acute appendicitis. *Ann Emerg Med.* 2004;44:S60.

Moore CL, Rose GA, Tayal VS et al. Determination of left ventricular function by emergency physician echocardiography of hypotensive patients. *Acad Emerg Med.* 2002;9(3):186–93.

Nagdev AD, Merchant RC, Tirado-Gonzalez A et al. Emergency department bedside ultrasonographic measurement of the caval index for noninvasive determination of low central venous pressure. *Ann Emerg Med.* 2010;55:290–5.

Nandipati KC, Allamaneni S, Kakarla R et al. Extended focused assessment with sonography for trauma (EFAST) in the diagnosis of pneumothorax: Experience at a community based level I trauma center. *Injury.* 2011;42:511–4.

Nelson M, Chiricolo G, Raio C et al. Can emergency physicians positively predict acute appendicitis on focused right lower quadrant ultrasound? *Ann Emerg Med.* 2005;46:27–8.

Nesselroade RD, Nickels LC. Ultrasound diagnosis of bilateral quadriceps tendon rupture after statin use. *West J Emerg Med.* 2010;11:306–9.

Ng C, Tsung JW. Avoiding computed tomography scans by using point-of-care ultrasound when evaluating suspected pediatric renal colic. *J Emerg Med.* 2015;49:165–71.

O'Malley M, Wilson S. Ultrasonography and computed tomography of appendicitis and diverticulitis. *Sem Roentgenol.* 2001;36:138–47.

O'Malley P, Tayal VS. Use of emergency musculoskeletal sonography in diagnosis of an open fracture of the hand. *J Ultrasound Med.* 2007;26:679–82.

Oshita R, Hunt M, Fox J et al. A retrospective analysis of the use of bedside ultrasonography in the diagnosis of acute appendicitis. *Ann Emerg Med.* 2004;44:S112.

Panebianco NL, Shofer F, Fields JM et al. The utility of transvaginal ultrasound in the ED evaluation of complications of first trimester pregnancy. *Am J Emerg Med.* 2015;33:743–8.

Plumb J, Mallin M, Bolte RG. The role of ultrasound in the emergency department evaluation of the acutely painful pediatric hip. *Pediatr Emerg Care.* 2015;31:54–8; quiz 9–61.

Plummer D, Brunnette D, Asinger R et al. Emergency department echocardiography improves outcome in penetrating cardiac injury. *Ann Emerg Med.* 1992;21:709–12.

Poortman P, Lohle PNM, Schoemaker CMC et al. Comparison of CT and sonography in the diagnosis of acute appendicitis. *AJR Am J Roentgenol.* 2003;181:1355–9.

Puylaert JB, Rutgers PH, Lalisang RI et al. A prospective study ultrasonography in the diagnosis of appendicitis. *N Engl J Med.* 1987;317:666–9.

Rosen CL, Brown DFM, Sagarin M et al. Ultrasonography by emergency physicians in detecting hydronephrosis in patients with suspected ureteral colic. *Acad Emerg Med.* 1996;3:541.

Ross M, Brown M, McLaughlin K et al. Emergency physician-performed ultrasound to diagnose cholelithiasis: A systematic review. *Acad Emerg Med.* 2011;18:227–35.

Roy S, Dewitz A, Paul I. Ultrasound-assisted ankle arthrocentesis. *Am J Emerg Med.* 1999;17:300–1.

Russell FM, Ehrman RR, Cosby K et al. Diagnosing acute heart failure in patients with undifferentiated dyspnea: A lung and cardiac ultrasound (LuCUS) protocol. *Acad Emerg Med.* 2015;22:182–91.

Shah VP, Tunik MG, Tsung JW. Prospective evaluation of point-of-care ultrasonography for the diagnosis of pneumonia in children and young adults. *JAMA Pediatr.* 2013;167:119–25.

Sheng AY, Dalziel P, Liteplo AS et al. Focused assessment with sonography in trauma and abdominal computed tomography utilization in adult trauma patients: Trends over the last decade. *Emerg Med Int.* 2013;2013:678380.

Siddiqui N, Arzola C, Friedman Z et al. Ultrasound improves cricothyrotomy success in cadavers with poorly defined neck anatomy: A randomized control trial. *Anesthesiology.* 2015;123:1033–41.

Sivitz AB, Cohen SG, Tejani C. Evaluation of acute appendicitis by pediatric emergency physician sonography. *Ann Emerg Med*. 2014;64:358–64.e4.

Smith-Bindman R, Aubin C, Bailitz J et al. Ultrasonography versus computed tomography for suspected nephrolithiasis. *N Engl J Med*. 2014;371:1100–10.

Sonosite iViz. 2016. Accessed May 7, 2017, at http://www.sonosite.com/sonosite-iviz.

Squire BT, Fox JC, Anderson C. ABSCESS: Applied bedside sonography for convenient evaluation of superficial soft tissue infections. *Acad Emerg Med*. 2005;12:601–6.

Stein JC, Wang R, Adler N et al. Emergency physician ultrasonography for evaluating patients at risk for ectopic pregnancy: A meta-analysis. *Ann Emerg Med*. 2010;56:674–83.

Summers SM, Scruggs W, Menchine MD et al. A prospective evaluation of emergency department bedside ultrasonography for the detection of acute cholecystitis. *Ann Emerg Med*. 2010;56:114–22.

Sutherland JE, Sutphin D, Redican K et al. Telesonography: Foundations and future directions. *J Ultrasound Med*. 2011;30:517–22.

Tayal VS, Bullard M, Swanson DR et al. ED endovaginal pelvic ultrasound in nonpregnant women with right lower quadrant pain. *Am J Emerg Med*. 2008;26:81–5.

Tayal VS, Graf CD, Gibbs, MA. Prospective study of accuracy and outcome of emergency ultrasound for abdominal aortic aneurysm over two years. *Acad Emerg Med*. 2003;10:867–71.

Tayal VS, Hasan N, Norton HJ et al. The effect of soft-tissue ultrasound on the management of cellulitis in the emergency department. *Acad Emerg Med*. 2006;13:384–8.

Tayal VS, Neulander M, Norton HJ et al. Emergency department sonographic measurement of optic nerve sheath diameter to detect findings of increased intracranial pressure in adult head injury patients. *Ann Emerg Med*. 2007;49:508–14.

Tayal VS, Nicks BA, Norton HJ. Emergency ultrasound evaluation of symptomatic nontraumatic pleural effusions. *Am J Emerg Med*. 2006;24:782–6.

Terasawa T, Blackmore CB, Bent S et al. Systematic review: Computed tomography and ultrasonography to detect acute appendicitis in adults and adolescents. *Ann Intern Med*. 2004;141:537–46.

Terasawa T, Hartling L, Cramer K, Klassen T. Diagnostic Accuracy of Ultrasound and Computed Tomography for Emergency Department Diagnosis of Appendicitis: A Systematic Review. *2nd International EM Conference 2003*.

Tessaro MO, Arroyo AC, Haines LE et al. Inflating the endotracheal tube cuff with saline to confirm correct depth using bedside ultrasonography. *CJEM*. 2015;17:94–8.

Vieira RL, Hsu D, Nagler J et al. Pediatric emergency medicine fellow training in ultrasound: Consensus educational guidelines. *Acad Emerg Med*. 2013;20:300–6.

Villar J, Summers SM, Menchine MD et al. The absence of gallstones on point-of-care ultrasound rules out acute cholecystitis. *J Emerg Med*. 2015;49:475–80.

Volpicelli G. Interpreting lung ultrasound B-lines in acute respiratory failure. *Chest*. 2014;146:e230.

Volpicelli G. Point-of-care lung ultrasound. *Praxis (Bern 1994)*. 2014;103:711–6.

Volpicelli G, Boero E, Sverzellati N et al. Semi-quantification of pneumothorax volume by lung ultrasound. *Intensive Care Med*. 2014;40:1460–7.

Volpicelli G, Zanobetti M. Lung ultrasound and pulmonary consolidations. *Am J Emerg Med*. 2015;33:1307–8.

Vrablik ME, Snead GR, Minnigan HJ et al. The diagnostic accuracy of bedside ocular ultrasonography for the diagnosis of retinal detachment: A systematic review and meta-analysis. *Ann Emerg Med*. 2015;65: 199–203.e1.

Weekes AJ, Reddy A, Lewis MR et al. E-point septal separation compared to fractional shortening measurements of systolic function in emergency department patients: Prospective randomized study. *J Ultrasound Med*. 2012;31:1891–7.

Weekes AJ, Tassone HM, Babcock A et al. Comparison of serial qualitative and quantitative assessments of caval index and left ventricular systolic function during early fluid resuscitation of hypotensive emergency department patients. *Acad Emerg Med*. 2011;18:912–21.

Zeidan BS, Wasser T, Nicholas GG. Ultrasonography in the diagnosis of acute appendicitis. *J R Coll Surg Edinb*. 1997;42:24–6.

Zieleskiewicz L, Muller L, Lakhal K et al. Point-of-care ultrasound in intensive care units: Assessment of 1073 procedures in a multicentric, prospective, observational study. *Intensive Care Med*. 2015;41:1638–47.

Index

A

Anisotropy, 204; *see also* Upper extremity nerve blocks
Ankle scanning, 75
 abscess overlying distal tibia, 78
 anterior view, 75, 76
 effusion, 78
 indications, 75
 normal, 77
 posterior placement of probe, 77
 posterior view, 75
 probe selection, 75
 talonavicular effusion, 79
 tibiotalar joint, 79
Appendicitis, 108, 109
 indications, 105
 maximal area of tenderness, 107
 ring of fire, 106
Appendix scanning, 105
 graded compression, 105
 probe selection, 105
 in sagittal orientation, 108
 in transverse orientation, 106, 107

B

Baker's cyst, 91; *see also* Soft-tissue scanning
Bile duct, 122; *see also* Biliary cholelithiasis scanning
 common, 122, 127–128
 dilated common, 128
 measurement, 124
Biliary cholelithiasis scanning, 121–122
 exclamation point sign, 123
 gallbladder wall measurement, 129
 gallstones, 125
 gallstone with posterior shadowing, 126
 indications, 121
 probe selection, 121
 sagittal orientation of probe in RUQ, 123
 sludge within gallbladder, 126
 WES SIGN, 127
Bladder scanning, 142, 143; *see also* Focused assessment sonography in trauma; Renal scanning
 stone view, 155
 in transverse orientation, 156
B lines; *see also* Pulmonary scanning
 within intercostal space, 27
 from pleura, 26
 in sagittal probe orientation, 26
Brachial plexus, 98; *see also* Neck scanning

Buckle fracture; *see also* Long bone scanning
   of radius, 41, 42
Bursitis, 57, 58; *see also* Elbow scanning

C

Cardiac scanning, 3
   apical four-chamber view, 7–8, 12
   indications, 3
   parasternal view, 4, 5, 8, 9, 10
   probe selection, 3
   subxiphoid view, 6–7, 11
Cellulitis, early, 86; *see also* Soft-tissue scanning
Central line placement, 207
   carotid view, 210
   indications, 207
   internal jugular vein view, 209–210
   probe selection, 207
   technique, 207–208
   views of femoral artery and vein, 211, 212
Cholelithiasis, 122; *see also* Biliary cholelithiasis scanning
Clavicle scanning, 43
   clavicle fracture, 47, 48
   indications, 43
   longitudinal orientation, 44–45, 46 , 47
   normal clavicle, 46
   probe selection, 43
   supra-clavicular notch, 44
   transverse orientation, 45, 46 , 47
Cobblestone, 86; *see also* Soft-tissue scanning
CRL, *see* Crown rump length
Crown rump length (CRL), 157
Cystic hygroma, 101; *see also* Neck scanning
Cyst in neck, 100

D

Displaced fracture, 37, 38, 39; *see also* Long bone scanning

E

Elbow scanning, 53
   anterior view, 53
   bursitis, 57, 58
   effusion, 59, 60
   fracture with overlying effusion, 60
   indications, 53
   joint effusion, 57
   normal elbow, 55
   posterior approach, 54
   posterior view, 53
   probe selection, 53
   transverse olecranon fossa, 56
Endotracheal tube confirmation, 189
   esophageal intubation, 191
   indications, 189
   probe selection, 189
   technique, 189
   tracheal ultrasound, 190
   transverse placement of probe on neck, 190
Enlarged lymph node, 100; *see also* Neck scanning
Exclamation point sign, 123; *see also* Biliary cholelithiasis scanning

Extraossous flow
    sagittal view, 182
    transverse view, 181
Eye, 218; *see also* Ocular scanning

F

Femoral nerve block scanning, 173–174
    contraindications, 173
    femoral nerve, 175
    femoral vein, 177–178
    indications, 173
    pre-procedure checklist, 173
    probe placement, 176
    probe selection, 173
Femoral nerve scanning
    distribution view, 175
    probe placement, 176
    transverse view of, 177
Femur bone, 37; *see also* Long bone scanning
Fetal heart rate (FHR), 157
FHR, *see* Fetal heart rate
Fluid pocket; *see also* Focused assessment sonography in trauma
    bladder, 142, 143
    at liver tip and in Morrison's pouch, 138
    at spleen tip, 140
    along sub-diaphragmatic space, 140
Focused assessment sonography in trauma (FAST), 21, 133
    anechoic free fluid pocket, 138
    bladder views, 142, 143
    cardiac view, 134
    fluid at spleen tip, 141
    fluid pocket, 140
    indications, 133
    normal LUQ view, 133–134, 139
    normal RUQ view, 133, 137, 138
    pericardial effusion, 136
    probe placement, 135, 139
    probe selection, 133
    subxiphoid view of heart, 136
    suprapubic view, 134, 141, 142
Foreign body, 90; *see also* Soft-tissue scanning
    hollow, 90
    linear, 89
    punctate, 89

G

Gallbladder wall measurement, 129; *see also* Biliary cholelithiasis scanning
Gallstones, 125; *see also* Biliary cholelithiasis scanning
    with posterior shadowing, 126
    sludge within, 126
Graded compression, 105; *see also* Appendix scanning; Intussusception
    lawnmower technique, 112

H

Hand nerve distribution, 201; *see also* Upper extremity nerve blocks
Hayfork sign, 114; *see also* Intussusception
Hip scanning, 61
    effusion, 64, 65, 66
    indications, 61

Hip scanning (*Continued*)
   in-plane evaluation, 64
   normal hip, 63
   probe in sagittal plane, 62
   probe selection, 61
Hydrocele scanning, 170; *see also* Testicular scanning
   in neonate, 169
Hydronephrosis; *see also* Renal scanning
   with hydroureter, 153, 154
   mild, 152, 153
   with renal parenchyma destruction, 155
   renal sinus destruction, 154

I

Inferior vena cava (IVC), 13
   collapse of, 17
   enlarged, 17
   entering right atrium, 16
   indications, 13
   longitudinal view of, 15
   probe placement, 14, 15
   probe selection, 13
   scanning, 13
   subxiphoid view, 13
   transverse axis view, 16
Internal jugular vein; *see also* Central line placement
   carotid, 210
   sagittal view, 210
   transverse view, 209–210
Intraosseous infusion, 181
Intraosseous placement, 179
   indications, 179
   probe in transverse orientation, 180
   probe selection, 179
   scanning, 179
   view of extraosseous flow, 181, 182
   view of intraosseous infusion, 180, 181
Intrauterine pregnancy (IUP), 157, 160, 161; *see also* Pregnancy scanning in first trimester
   with hyperechoic ring, 163
   view of uterus with, 161
   view of uterus without, 162
Intussusception, 111
   graded compression technique, 113
   Hayfork sign, 114
   indications, 111
   lawnmower technique, 112
   probe selection, 111
   transverse view, 113, 115
   wall-to-wall measurement, 114
IUP, *see* Intrauterine pregnancy
IVC, *see* Inferior vena cava

K

Kidney, 151, 152, 153; *see also* Renal scanning
Knee scanning, 67
   anatomical features, 68
   anterior view of, 68
   indications, 67
   normal, 72
   prepatellar bursitis, 74
   prepatellar septic bursitis, 73
   probe placement, 69, 70, 71
   probe selection, 67
   quadriceps tendon rupture, 72
   quadriceps tendon rupture with hematoma, 73

L

Left upper quadrant (LUQ), 133–134
Long bone scanning, 35
 displaced fracture, 37, 38, 39
 femur, 37
 indications, 35
 probe selection, 35
 radius, 36, 41
 radius fracture, 41, 42
 rib fracture, 39
 tibia, 37, 39, 40
Lumbar puncture, 183
 indications, 183
 probe placement, 184
 probe selection, 183
 sagittal orientation, 185
 technique, 183
 transverse orientation, 186
 view of spinous processes, 185, 187
Lung, 28–29; *see also* Pulmonary scanning
 pneumonia consolidation, 31
 lung point sign, 30–31
 sagittal probe orientation, 25
LUQ, *see* Left upper quadrant
Lymph nodes, 96, 99; *see also* Neck scanning
 in anterior cervical chain, 99
 enlarged lymph node, 100
 intussusception with entrapped, 115

M

Mac-off retinal detachment, 216, 221; *see also* Ocular scanning
Mac-on retinal detachments, 216; *see also* Ocular scanning
Median nerve, 202, 203; *see also* Upper extremity nerve blocks
 block, 200
 in mid-forearm, 204

N

Neck scanning, 93
 arterial and venous vasculature, 95
 brachial plexus, 98
 cystic hygroma, 101
 cyst in, 100
 fluctuant mass on, 97
 indications, 93
 lymph nodes, 96, 99, 100
 patient positioning, 94
 probe placement, 94
 probe selection, 93
 scanning, 93
 sublingual glands, 96
 submandibular gland abscess, 101
 view of thyroid and trachea, 97
Nerve; *see also* Upper extremity nerve blocks
 distribution in hand, 201
 median nerve, 202, 203
 radial artery and, 206
 radial nerve, 202
 ulnar artery and, 205
 ulnar nerve, 203

O

Ocular scanning, 215, 219
 indications, 215

Ocular scanning (*Continued*)
  normal eye, 218
  normal vitreous, 218
  optic nerve sheath measurement, 215–216, 220
  papilledema, 222
  posterior vitreous detachments, 216
  probe placement, 217
  probe selection, 215
  retinal detachment, 216, 221
  retinoblastoma, 222

P

Papilledema, 222; *see also* Ocular scanning
Pericardial effusion, 136; *see also* Focused assessment sonography in trauma
Peripheral intravenous placement, 193
  confirmation of needle within vein, 196
  indications, 193
  peripheral line confirmation, 197
  peripheral vein with IV, 198
  probe placement, 194
  probe selection, 193
  transverse view of needle, 197
  veins with tourniquet, 195
Peripheral vein, 195, 196
Pleura evaluation, abnormal, 30; *see also* Pulmonary scanning
Pleural effusion, 21–22; *see also* Pulmonary scanning
Pneumonia; *see also* Pulmonary scanning
  with air bronchograms, 32
  lung consolidation, 31
Pneumothorax, 29; *see also* Pulmonary scanning
Posterior vitreous detachments, 216; *see also* Ocular scanning
Pregnancy scanning in first trimester, 157
  hyperechoic ring, 163
  indications, 157
  intrauterine pregnancy, 160, 161
  probe placement, 159
  probe selection, 157
  transabdominal, 157
  transvaginal, 158
  view of intrauterine pregnancy, 162
  view of uterus, 159, 160, 161
  yolk sac, 162
Prepatellar bursitis, 74; *see also* Knee scanning
Prepatellar septic bursitis, 73; *see also* Knee scanning
Pulmonary scanning, 21
  abnormal pleura evaluation, 30
  B lines from pleura, 26
  B lines in sagittal probe orientation, 26
  B lines within intercostal space, 27
  consolidation, 31
  indications, 21
  lung point sign, 30–31
  normal lung, 25, 28–29
  pleural effusion, 21–22
  pneumonia, 31
  pneumothorax, 29
  probe selection, 21
  right upper quadrant view, 27, 28
  transducer placement, 22, 23, 24

Pylorus, 117
   indications, 117
   probe placement, 118
   probe selection, 117
   scanning, 117
   transverse view, 119
   view of hypertrophic, 119
Pyomyositis, 88; *see also* Soft-tissue scanning

Q

Quadriceps tendon rupture; *see also* Knee scanning
   with hematoma, 73
   in sagittal plane, 72

R

Radial artery, 206; *see also* Upper extremity nerve blocks
Radial nerve, 202, 206; *see also* Upper extremity nerve blocks
   block, 199
Renal scanning, 147
   bladder in transverse orientation, 155, 156
   hydronephrosis with hydroureter, 154
   hydronephrosis with renal parenchyma destruction, 155
   hydronephrosis with renal sinus destruction, 154
   indications, 147
   mild hydronephrosis, 152, 153
   moderate hydronephrosis with hydroureter, 153
   probe placement, 148, 149, 150
   probe selection, 147
   view of kidney, 151, 152, 153
   visualization of right kidney, 150
Retinal detachment, 216, 221; *see also* Ocular scanning
Retinoblastoma, 222; *see also* Ocular scanning
Right upper quadrant (RUQ), 133
Ring of fire, 106; *see also* Appendix scanning
RUQ, *see* Right upper quadrant

S

Shoulder scanning, 49
   hematoma block, 52
   indications, 49
   posterior view, 49
   probe selection, 49
   shoulder joint effusion, 51
   view at glenohumeral joint, 51
Soft-tissue scanning, 83
   abscess, 87, 91
   baker's cyst, 91
   cobblestone, 86
   early cellulitis, 86
   foreign body, 89, 90
   indications, 83
   normal soft tissue, 85
   probe orientation, 84, 85
   probe selection, 83
   pyomyositis, 88
   thigh hematoma, 88
Spinous processes, 185, 187; *see also* Lumbar puncture
Sublingual glands, 96; *see also* Neck scanning
Submandibular gland abscess, 101; *see also* Neck scanning

T

Talonavicular effusion, 79; *see also* Ankle scanning
Testicular scanning, 165, 166
  hydrocele, 169, 170
  indications, 165
  normal testicles, 166, 167
  probe selection, 165
  testicles with increased flow, 167
  testicles with no flow, 168
  testicular torsion, 168, 169
Thigh hematoma, 88; *see also* Soft-tissue scanning
Tibia bone, 37; *see also* Long bone scanning
  fracture of, 39, 40
  normal, 40
Tibiotalar joint, 79; *see also* Ankle scanning
Transverse olecranon fossa, 56; *see also* Elbow scanning

U

Ulnar artery, 205; *see also* Upper extremity nerve blocks
Ulnar nerve, 203; *see also* Upper extremity nerve blocks
  block, 199–200
Upper extremity nerve blocks, 199
  anisotropy, 204
  indications, 199
  median nerve, 202, 203, 204
  median nerve block, 200
  nerve distribution in hand, 201
  probe selection, 199
  radial artery, 206
  radial nerve, 202, 206
  radial nerve block, 199
  scanning, 199
  ulnar artery, 205
  ulnar nerve, 203, 205
  ulnar nerve block, 199–200
Uterus, 159, 160, 161, 162; *see also* Pregnancy scanning in first trimester

V

Vitreous, 218; *see also* Ocular scanning
  detachment, 216

W

WES SIGN, 127; *see also* Biliary cholelithiasis scanning

Y

Yolk sac, 162; *see also* Pregnancy scanning in first trimester

For Product Safety Concerns and Information please contact our EU representative GPSR@taylorandfrancis.com Taylor & Francis Verlag GmbH, Kaufingerstraße 24, 80331 München, Germany

Printed and bound by CPI Group (UK) Ltd, Croydon, CR0 4YY
08/06/2025
01896985-0001